Case Studies in

PHYSIOLOGY
and
NUTRITION

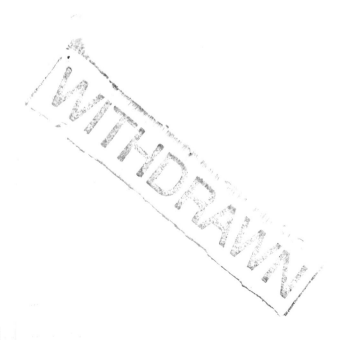

Case Studies in

PHYSIOLOGY
and
NUTRITION

Lynne Berdanier • Carolyn D. Berdanier

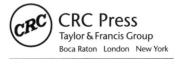

CRC Press
Taylor & Francis Group
Boca Raton   London   New York

CRC Press is an imprint of the
Taylor & Francis Group, an **informa** business

CRC Press
Taylor & Francis Group
6000 Broken Sound Parkway NW, Suite 300
Boca Raton, FL 33487-2742

© 2010 by Taylor and Francis Group, LLC
CRC Press is an imprint of Taylor & Francis Group, an Informa business

No claim to original U.S. Government works

Printed in the United States of America on acid-free paper
10 9 8 7 6 5 4 3 2 1

International Standard Book Number: 978-1-4200-8877-9 (Paperback)

Library of Congress Cataloging-in-Publication Data

Berdanier, Lynne.
    Case studies in physiology and nutrition / Lynne Berdanier, Carolyn D. Berdanier.
        p. ; cm.
    Includes index.
    ISBN 978-1-4200-8877-9 (pbk. : alk. paper)
    1. Clinical biochemistry--Case studies. 2. Nutritionally induced diseases--Case studies. I. Berdanier, Carolyn D. II. Title.
    [DNLM: 1. Nutritional Physiological Phenomena--Problems and Exercises. 2. Homeostasis--Problems and Exercises. 3. Nutritional and Metabolic Diseases--Problems and Exercises. QU 18.2 B486c 2010]

    RB112.5.B47 2010
    616.07--dc22   2009027560

Visit the Taylor & Francis Web site at
http://www.taylorandfrancis.com

and the CRC Press Web site at
http://www.crcpress.com

Contents

Chapter 1 How to Use This Book 1
What Is a Case Study? 1
Sample Case Study: Derrick's Malaise...2
Where Can I Find the Answers to These Problems? 3
Where Does the Analysis Part Come In?..3
    Key Words and Their Meanings: Look Up the Unfamiliar Terms 3
    Read the Relevant Literature 3
    Organize Your Information 4
    Prepare a Summary for Yourself of the Previous Key Points......................4
What Do the Terms Used in This Book Mean?..4
Learning Activity 1.1 8
Learning Activity 1.2 9

Chapter 2 Disease 11
What Is a Disease? 11
How Is Disease Studied? Who Studies Disease? 12
Do We Keep Track of Disease? 12
What Causes a Disease to Develop?..12
What Are Signs and Symptoms? 13
What Kinds of Laboratory Work Could Be Helpful in Describing the Case?.....13
What Kinds of Tissues Can Be Used for Laboratory Assessment?.....................14
How Long Does a Disease Last? 14
Learning Activity 2.1: Epidemiology Case Study 16
    Suspected Legionnaires' Disease in Bogalusa..16
        The Story 16
        Background on Bogalusa..17
        Conclusion 19

Chapter 3 Homeostasis 21
What Is Homeostasis? 21
How Is Homeostasis Regulated? 21
What Is the Relevance of Homeostatic Control to Our Understanding of the
Physiology of Nutrition? 23
Malnutrition as Part of a Homeostatic Disturbance 24
    Sodium...25
    Potassium 26
    Chloride 26

Calcium..27
Magnesium...28
Other Instances of Homeostatic Regulation 28
Growth and Development 28
Obesity 28
Homeostasis in Body Weight Regulation..30
Treatment of Obesity 30
Drugs in the Treatment of Obesity 31
Diet Products 31
Bariatric Surgery 32
Conclusion..33
Learning Activity 3.1: Keeping a Food Diary 34
Case Study 3.1: Marcus Wants to Stop Gaining Weight........................35
Problem Analysis and Resolution...36
Case Study 3.2: Susie's Goldfish Jumps Out of the Bowl.....................37
Problem Analysis and Resolution...37
Case Study 3.3: Beth Decides..38
Problem Analysis and Resolution...38
Case Study 3.4: Baby Bo Can't Get Enough 40
Problem Analysis and Resolution...40
Case Study 3.5: Discovering a Concentration Camp 42
Problem Analysis and Resolution...42

Chapter 4   Blood...**43**
Causes of Nutritional Anemia 43
Pharmacological Treatment of Iron Deficiency 46
Toxicology of Iron Overload 46
Other Nutrients and Anemia...47
Non-Nutritional Anemia..48
Blood Groups...48
Blood Clotting..49
White Cells...50
Blood Pressure...51
Learning Activity 4.1: Your Nutritional Status.....................................53
Case Study 4.1: Cynthia Has an Automobile Accident..........................54
Problem Analysis and Resolution...54
Case Study 4.2: Nebraska Pioneer Women..55
Problem Analysis and Resolution...55
Case Study 4.3: Maureen Decides to Adopt Vegetarianism 56
Problem Analysis and Resolution...56

Chapter 5   You Are What You Eat..**57**
Dietary Guidelines..57
Diet Assessment..57
Nutritional Assessment...61
Laboratory Tests..62
Case Study 5.1: Elise Complains of Trouble Driving at Night.............64
Problem Analysis and Resolution...64

Case Study 5.2: Uncle John Is an Alcoholic 65
  Problem Analysis and Resolution...65
Case Study 5.3: Little Lizzie Has Scurvy 66
  Problem Analysis and Resolution...66

Chapter 6   How Is Food Used? 67
How Do We Get the Nutrients in the Food into Our Bodies? 67
Absorption 67
Protein Digestion 68
Amino Acid Absorption 69
Carbohydrate Digestion 69
Carbohydrate Absorption 71
Lipid Digestion and Absorption 71
Case Study 6.1: Steven Has a Belly Ache 75
  Problem Analysis and Resolution...75
Case Study 6.2: John Has a Pain...76
  Problem Analysis and Resolution...76
Case Study 6.3: Emily's Baby 77
  Problem Analysis and Resolution...77
Case Study 6.4: Herbert Is on a Food Supplement Kick 78
  Problem Analysis and Resolution...78
Case Study 6.5: Herman Is Convinced He Has Heart Trouble..........................79
  Problem Analysis and Resolution...79

Chapter 7   We Are What We Inherit 81
What Is a Gene? What Is Our Genotype? What Is Our Phenotype? What Is the
Difference between the Terms, Genotype and Phenotype? 81
How Do We Inherit Our Genotype and Phenotype? 83
How Does Our Environment Shape the Phenotypic Expression of Our Genotype? 84
Learning Activity 7.1: Your Family Tree 88
Case Study 7.1: An African Adventure 89
  Problem Analysis and Resolution...89
Case Study 7.2: BoBo Hates Milk; It Gives Him a Tummy Ache......................90
  Problem Analysis and Resolution...90
Case Study 7.3: Sylvia, Raymond, and Reginald Have a Fat Mother with
Type 2 Diabetes 91
  Problem Analysis and Resolution...91

Chapter 8   Pets and People..93
How the Immune System Works 93
Antibodies...95
Types of Diseases of the Immune System 96
Case Study 8.1: The Horse with the Flying Tail...98
  Problem Analysis and Resolution...98
Case Study 8.2: Chuck Has a Parakeet...99
  Problem Analysis and Resolution...99
Case Study 8.3: Elizabeth Has a Dog Problem..100
  Problem Analysis and Resolution...100

Case Study 8.4: Betty Changes Allegiances 101
    Problem Analysis and Resolution 101
Case Study 8.5: Julia Is Thin 102
    Problem Analysis and Resolution 102

Chapter 9   Food and Health **103**
Food Safety 103
Food-Borne Pathogens 103
    Bacteria 103
    Viruses 105
    Eukaryotic Contaminants (Molds and Parasites) 106
Recognition 106
Prevention 106
Case Study 9.1: Traveler's Tummy 107
    Problem Analysis and Resolution 107
Case Study 9.2: Oh Those Tomatoes! 109
    Problem Analysis and Resolution 109
Case Study 9.3: Jesse and His Family Get Sick 110
    Problem Analysis and Resolution 110

Chapter 10 Stones and Bones **111**
Bone Mineralization 111
Bone Diseases 111
    Osteoporosis 113
    Osteomalacia 114
Skeletal Problems Associated with Renal Disease 114
Other Diseases of the Bone 114
Renal Stone Disease 115
    Types of Stones 115
Case Study 10.1: Aunt Tillie Is Getting Shorter 117
    Problem Analysis and Resolution 117
Case Study 10.2: Mike Writhes on the Floor 118
    Problem Analysis and Resolution 118
Case Study 10.3: Bertha Takes a Fall 119
    Problem Analysis and Resolution 119

Chapter 11 Age and Nutrition **121**
The Aging Process 121
Age-Related Changes in Metabolism 123
Case Study 11.1: Grandma Is Tired 125
    Problem Analysis and Resolution 125
Case Study 11.2: Lydia Has Palpitations 126
    Problem Analysis and Resolution 126

Chapter 12 Getting from Here to There—Muscle **127**
Types of Muscle and Their Function 127
How Nutrition Affects Muscle Function 129
Muscle Problems 130
Learning Activity 12.1: Your Basal Energy Need 131

Learning Activity 12.2: Activity Cost.. 132
Learning Activity 12.3: Exploring Performance-Enhancing Products 134
Case Study 12.1: Jason Is a Cyclist 135
    Problem Analysis and Resolution.. 135
Case Study 12.2: Jackson Aspires to Play Professional Football 136
    Problem Analysis and Resolution.. 136
Case Study 12.3: Tonya Has a Heart Attack 137
    Problem Analysis and Resolution.. 137
Case Study 12.4: Edward Enlists in the Army 138
    Problem Analysis and Resolution.. 138

Glossary 139

Index 149

Preface

Today's knowledge of human health demands a multidisciplinary understanding of medically related sciences. This volume is dedicated to the integration of nutrition science with physiology. It is written using descriptions of human problems so as to stimulate the student's thinking about the body and how it works.

Each of the case studies presented has a physiological approach, and it is expected that the student will use this approach in his/her discussion of the disorder and the strategies that will help resolve the disorder. These problems are not medical exercises, nor are they intended to simulate medical training. They are, however, exercises designed to stimulate the student to think about how the body integrates various physiological factors to maintain homeostasis.

Since the problems presented here are meant to integrate many avenues of health science, it is anticipated that more than one resource will be needed to answer the problems completely. In most cases the student will want to develop a strategy for resolving the problem. Some of the cases are very straightforward with very simple answers, while others will require in-depth thinking and literature searching to resolve.

A "disease" approach has been used in describing each of the cases. That is, a story has been created to describe a real-life situation that might be something to which a student could relate. The student is asked to use multiple resources (books, libraries, Internet data sources, etc.) to explain what is happening in the body and why the case developed. The student is then asked to develop strategies based on principles of physiology and nutrition that will alleviate the situation. It is hoped that the student will develop critical thinking skills through these exercises.

Acknowledgments

The authors would like to express their appreciation to their families for their support and patience as this book was prepared. This book would not have been possible without the gracious encouragement of our editor, Randy Brehm, of the Taylor & Francis Group. Lynne would also like to thank Jean E. Miller, Joan S. Griffith, and Michelle Barth for past firmness of character, and RSM for being himself. Last, the authors would like to thank our colleagues who read the manuscript. We thank Thomas Nelson, Frances Kennedy, Ryan Shanks, Kimberly Shanks, Stephanie Songer, and H. Keith Brown for their gracious contributions of their time and expertise.

About the Authors

Lynne Berdanier teaches anatomy and physiology in the Department of Biology at North Georgia College and State University in Dahlonega, Georgia. Prior to teaching in Dahlonega she taught at Athens Technical College in Athens, Georgia. She earned an MS in physiology from the University of Georgia and had further graduate study at the University of Missouri. She has authored laboratory manuals for medical microbiology and for anatomy and physiology. In addition, she has had considerable experience in industry with respect to biotechnology. She is listed in *Who's Who in American Teaching* and has several publications in the biochemistry/physiology field.

Carolyn Berdanier has had a long and productive career in nutrition. She began her career as a nutrition scientist with U.S. Department of Agriculture in Beltsville, Maryland. At the same time she served as a faculty member with the University of Maryland. After this, she served on the faculty of the University of Nebraska College of Medicine, and following that moved to the University of Georgia. Her research into nutrient–gene interactions and in mitochondrial function was supported by a variety of agencies. Her publication record is extensive. She has served on a number of editorial boards and study sections. She has been recognized for her research contributions with a variety of awards including outstanding alumna awards from Rutgers and the Pennsylvania State University, the Lamar Dodd Award for Creative Research, the UGA Research Medal, the National 4-H Award for Alumni, and the Borden Award from AHEA, and she was elected a Fellow in the American Society for Nutrition Science.

was sitting in the waiting room wondering if he could contract malaria from Derrick. What problems do you see in this case study?

First, what is malaria? Look this up. Look up the common treatments and also look up how the disease is carried. This will answer the question that Derrick's roommate has about whether he is at risk for developing the disease. Then, look to see whether there are any nutritional implications in this case. Would Derrick's nutritional status have affected his vulnerability to malaria? Would the drugs used for the treatment of malaria have any interaction with certain nutrients? Do a search on drug–nutrient interactions. It could be quite revealing. Last, look up the responses to quinine drugs. Find out how they work. Also find out whether all people can take them. Ask whether there are some genetically dictated differences in the responses to these drugs.

Where Can I Find the Answers to These Problems?

Begin by finding out what the case is about. Read through the case to get a sense of the problem you are facing. If you are working in a group, have one person read the case aloud and then individually make a list of all the unknown terms, the system(s) involved, and the key bits of information.

Where Does the Analysis Part Come In?

Analysis happens when you and/or your group begin to ask questions about the case. Some of the questions will be simple, others complex. Some will involve unfamiliar terms and their meanings. Look them up. Other questions will evolve as you delve into the literature about the case you are studying. Usually, case study analysis involves four steps:

Key Words and Their Meanings: Look Up the Unfamiliar Terms

Example of questions that might occur to you in the case of Derrick's malaise:

1. What is this case about?
2. Malaria: What is it? How is it caused? What are its symptoms?
3. Why may it reoccur?
4. How is it treated?
5. How is it transmitted?

Read the Relevant Literature

Try to find the answers to the following questions:

1. How do malarial drugs work?
2. Why did Derrick have a relapse?
3. Look up the U.S. incidence and prevalence of malaria.
4. Look up the worldwide rates of malarial infections.
5. What are the optimal conditions for disease transmission?
6. What is The Centers for Disease Control? How does it act as a monitoring agency of U.S. and global disease health problems?

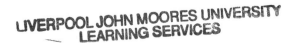

You might even want to ask yourself what further laboratory measurements might help you accept or decline the solutions that will emerge as you think about the case.

Organize Your Information

Again, using the previous example you might want to make a table listing on one side what you know or have found out about malaria, its treatment, and its effects on the body and on the other side list what more you need to learn in order to finish your analysis of the case.

Prepare a Summary for Yourself of the Previous Key Points

Submit this summary to your team if you are working in a team and then prepare a summary for your instructor.

While some of the case studies in this book are quite simple, others are not. You will need to understand all of the ways the body is working (or failing to work) in order to understand the problem. You will need to go to texts of physiology as well as nutrition texts to find all the information you will need to prepare your responses. Use the Web as a source of information but be careful to use only Web sites that are written by knowledgeable people and refereed. Table 1.1 gives examples of useful Web sites. There are many to choose from. You can Google key words from your case study to obtain good sources of information such as those prepared by the National Institutes of Health (Medline). Avoid the use of Web sites created by and for the lay reader. Some of the information may not be correct and/or current. Some might contain undocumented and untested material.

Some of the cases may seem straightforward but as you delve into the problem you will discover they are not so simple after all. Stretch your imagination and give it your best creative thought. Don't forget that some of these cases have social, cultural, and/or economic overtones that need to be explored. Your solutions and strategies should relate to the whole picture not just to the immediate problem.

What Do the Terms Used in This Book Mean?

Many of the terms are clinical terms and their definitions can be found in a medical dictionary. There are several on the market, and your library will probably have them on its shelves. For example, *Stedman's Medical Dictionary* published by Williams & Wilkins, and updated at regular intervals, is an excellent source of information on medical terms. *Dorman's Medical Dictionary* and several others are good examples. The *CRC Desk Reference for Nutrition* by Berdanier (C.D. Berdanier, 2nd edition, 2006, Taylor & Francis, Boca Raton FL) is also a good source of information.

There are a number of prefixes and suffixes that are in common use in medical terms. Some prefixes are listed in Table 1.2. Understanding their use can help you understand the symptom being described. As examples, the prefix *hyper-* means that the value given is above normal, while the prefix *hypo-* means that the value is below normal. The prefix *poly-* means many or excess. *Polyuria* means excess urination or large volumes of urine being produced. *Polydipsia* means excessive water consumption. There are other terms that one should remember as well: *Fasting* means that no food has been consumed for at least 8 hours. Sometimes fasting is used to indicate longer periods of time without food. If the individual is without food for 24 hours or more, then the person is starving. Fasting and starvation can be either voluntary or involuntary. In the latter case, it is usually because no

Table 1.2 Prefixes Used in Medical Terms

Prefix	Example	Meaning
Pre- (before)	Prenatal	Period before birth
Peri- (around)	Perinatal	Period around birth
Epi- (above, upon)	Epidermis	Outer most layer of skin
Hypo- (under, below)	Hypodermic	Under the skin
Hyper- (above)	Hyperglycemic	Above normal blood sugar
Infra- (under, below)	Infracostal	Below the ribs
Sub- (under, below)	Subdural	Below the dura mater
Inter- (between)	Intercostal	Between the ribs
Post- (behind)	Posterior	Back part of anatomical point
Retro- (backward, behind)	Retroversion	Tipping backward
Bi- (two)	Bilateral	Two sides
Diplo- (two)	Diplococcus	Two attached bacterial cells
Hemi- (one-half)	Hemiplegia	Paralysis of one body side
Macro- (large)	Macrophage	Large cell
Micro- (small)	Microscope	Instrument for magnification
Ab- (from, away from)	Abduction	Movement away from center line of body
Ad- (toward)	Adduction	Movement toward center line of body
Circum- (around)	Circumduction	Movement in a circular direction
A- (without, not)	Aphagic	Not eating
Anti- (against)	Antibacterial	Against bacteria
Contra- (not)	Contraindicted	Not recommended
Brady- (slow)	Bradycardia	Slow heart rate
Tachy- (rapid)	Tachycardia	Rapid heart rate
Dys- (bad, painful)	Dystocia	Difficult childbirth
Homeo- (same)	Homeostasis	Maintenance of sameness
Eu- (good, normal)	Eupnea	Normal breathing
Mal- (bad)	Malnutrition	Any disturbance in adequate intakes of nutrients
Pseudo- (false)	Pseudostratified	False appearance of cell layers

food is available for consumption or the individual is unable to eat. *Prandial* means after a meal; *preprandial* means just before a meal. The term *hyperphagia* means excess eating that occurs beyond the eating that meets the nutrient needs of the individual. *Hypophagia* is the reverse. This is when a person does not eat sufficient food to meet his/her biological need for nutrients. *Aphagia* is when the individual eats little or nothing and is essentially starving. *Plasma* is what is left from blood after all the formed elements (red and white blood cells and platelets) have been removed. *Serum* is what is left from blood after the clotting factors have been removed. Last, the term *normal* means that the value (or range of values) is what is found in apparently healthy individuals. Tables 1.3, 1.4, and 1.5 give normal values for components in blood and other fluids. Usually these values are from adult individuals. Some gender and age differences are known and where possible these are indicated. Normal values or ranges of values are shown in the tables for blood and urine.

As you are reading the case studies presented in this book, look at the terminology being used. It may give you clues as to the condition of the individual being described. If you do not know what the terms mean, look them up. Likewise, if you do not understand

Table 1.3 Normal Values for Blood

Measurement	Normal Range of Values
Red blood cells (million/cu mm)	Males: 4.6–6.2; Females: 4.2–5.4
Hemoglobin (g/dl)	Males: 14–18; Females: 12–16
Hematocrit (vol %)	Males: 40–54%; Females: 37–47%
Serum iron (ug/dl)	60–280
TIBC[a] (ug/dl)	250–425
Ferritin (ng/ml)	Males: 30–300; Females: 20–120
Microcytes	Few
Macrocytes	Few
Red cell folate (nmol/l)	>360
Serum folate (mg/ml)	>13.5
Serum B_{12} (pg/ml)	200–900
MCV[b] (cu m)	82–92

[a] Total iron binding capacity; this is an indirect measure of serum transferrin.
[b] Mean cell volume.

Table 1.4 Other Constituents in Blood

Constituent	Normal Range of Values
Cholesterol, total (mg/dL)	100–199
Triglycerides (mg/dL)	0–149
HDL cholesterol (mg/dL)	40–59
VLDL cholesterol (calc., mg/dL)	5–40
LDL cholesterol (calc., mg/dL)	0–99
Hemoglobin A1C (%)[a]	4.8–5.9
Glucose (mg/dL)	75–109
Urea nitrogen (mg/dL)	5–26
Serum creatinine (mg/dL)	0.5–1.5
Serum sodium (mmol/dL)	135–145
Serum potassium (mmol/dL)	3.5–5.2
Serum chloride (mmol/dL)	97–108
Carbon dioxide (mmol/L)	20–32
Calcium (mg/dL)	8.5–10.6
Protein (g/dL)	6–8.5
Albumin (g/dL)	3.5–4.8
Globulin (g/dL)	1.5–4.5
Bilirubin (mg/dL)	0.1–1.2
Alkaline phosphatase (IU/L)	25–165
AST (SGOT)[b] (IU/L)	0–40
ALT (SGPT)[b] (IU/L)	0–40
Creatine kinase[c] (IU/L)	10–50
Lactate dehydrogenase (IU/L)	55–140

[a] This is a measure of the long-term blood glucose levels and is used to monitor glucose homeostasis.
[b] This is a measure of transaminase activity and is an indicator of tissue damage as in a damaged muscle.
[c] Myokinase and creatine kinase activity are indicators of heart tissue damage.

Table 1.5 Normal Laboratory Values for Clinical Assessments

Constituent	Range of Normal Values
Acetone, Acetoacetate (S)	0.3–2 mg/dL (3–20 mg/L)
Aldosterone (U)	2–26 ug/24 hours
Ammonia (P)	10–80 ug/dL
Catecholamines, total (U)	Less than 100 ug/24 hours
Cortisol (U)	20–100 ug/24 hours
Amylase (S)	80–180 units/dL
Bicarbonate (S)	24–28 meq/L
Ceruloplasmin(S)	25–43 mg/dL (1.7–2.9 μmol/L)
γ-Glutamyl transpeptidase (S)	Less than 30 units/L
Lactate (B)	4–16 mg/dL (0.44–1.8 mmol/L)
Phospholipid (S)	145–200 mg/dL (1.45–2 g/dL)
Pyruvate (B)	0.6–1 mg/dL (70–114 umol/L)
Serotonin (B)	5–20 ug/dL

Abbreviations used: S, serum; U, urine; B, whole blood; P, plasma

the systems involved, look these up as well. As you search for understanding you will learn a lot about the physiology of nutrition and what normal physiology can be expected in healthy individuals. This in turn will help you understand the role of nutrition in the health and welfare of all living creatures. There are many species similarities (and some differences too!) that when considered all together help us understand the basic biochemistry and physiology of the living world.

Learning Activity 1.1

Place a slash after each of the following prefixes and then define the prefix. The first one has been completed for you.

Word	Definition of Prefix
Inter/cellular	___between cells_____
Hypodermic	_____
Hypoxia	_____
Hypercalcemia	_____
Subdermal	_____
Retrograde fever	_____
Sublingual	_____
Transdermal	_____
Polydipsia	_____
Intramuscular	_____
Ataxia	_____
Apnea	_____
Malabsorption	_____
Pseudopod	_____

Learning Activity 1.2

Match the following terms with the definitions in the numbered list.

Abiotic   Dystocia

Antibacterial   Homosexual

Bradycardia   Tachycardia

Contraception   Postprandial

1._____ rapid heartbeat

2._____ against bacteria

3._____ pertaining to the same sex

4._____ no fertilization of an egg by sperm (no embryo is formed)

5._____ slow heart rate

6._____ no life

7._____ difficult or painful childbirth

8._____ after eating

chapter 2

Disease

What Is a Disease?

The maintenance of internal sameness is called *homeostasis*. If this maintenance is perturbed by either external factors or internal ones, then a disease state may develop. So, what is disease? Disease is any deviation from normal that interferes with body function. Disease may be resolved by recovery, partial recovery (now referred to as a chronic disease that can be managed), or death. Disease produces signs and symptoms noticeable by laboratory tests and/or by physical examination. Signs are objective, measurable evidence of a deviation from normal. A sign might be an abnormal pulse or heart rate or an elevated body temperature. Symptoms are indicators of disease that are overlaid with patient perceptions such as pain, dizziness, and itching. The case studies in this book all use signs and symptoms as a means of indicating the possible physiological cause for the problem being discussed.

Disease will usually have a traceable causative factor. This is called the *etiology* of the disease. The process of disease development is called the *pathophysiology* of that disease. It includes not only the progression of signs and symptoms but can also include causative factors such as exposure to a pathogen, the phenotypic expression of a particular genotype, and exposure to a toxin. The term *disease* can also include those deviations from normal that occur through injury as in an automobile accident. Accidents may involve the skeletal system but could also be due to unexpected exposure to fire (burns), chemical spills, and so forth. As can be seen, deviation from normal homeostasis can occur in a variety of circumstances. The challenge for healthcare professionals is to identify what caused the deviation from normal in the individual under their care. Many disease states can be identified through a careful examination of the presenting signs and symptoms. However, other situations might require inquiry into the working and/or living environment or the social/cultural environment and the choice of activities that might have preceded this deviation from normal. A family medical history might be informative as well.

Some individuals are genetically susceptible to diseases such as diabetes while others are not. The same is true for susceptibility to other degenerative diseases such as heart disease, renal disease, and obesity. Genetic factors as well can interact with environmental factors, and in turn these interactions can determine whether a specific disease will develop. For example, if an individual is genetically susceptible to obesity yet lives in an environment where food is in short supply and the individual must exert considerable energy to obtain both food and other necessities of living, then that individual will not become obese. Another example: If the person is genetically susceptible to lactose intolerance but never consumes milk, then the symptoms of lactose intolerance will not develop.

Last, there are also age-related degenerative diseases such as coronary vessel disease, which is thought to be related to elevated levels of cholesterol in the blood. Prolonged elevated serum cholesterol levels can result in a deposition of sterols and other substances on the walls of the vascular tree. This is known as plaque. When a plaque occurs and grows, vessel blockages develop. This means that the tissues served by the blocked vessel do not receive sufficient oxygen and are unable to have their toxic wastes removed by the blood that usually supplies that tissue. The part of the tissue served by that vessel may die. If the vessel is tiny or in some peripheral part of the body, this damage is not as serious as happens when a major vessel of the heart or the brain or some other vital organ is affected. This disease is called *atherosclerosis* or *arteriosclerosis*. Both genetic factors and dietary factors are involved in the pathophysiology of this disease.

How Is Disease Studied? Who Studies Disease?

Many different disciplines study disease from a variety of perspectives. An anthropologist, for example, studies disease patterns in population groups to determine what factors are common or uncommon in afflicted versus unafflicted individuals. A public health worker studies disease patterns for much the same reasons, but the public health worker is interested in finding predictors of the disease and effectiveness of treatments from a population perspective. A nutrition scientist might study the pathophysiology of a disease to determine whether nutritional status is involved or whether specific nutrients are implicated. Physicians study the disease from a treatment perspective. They want to know what the best treatment might be to cure the disease or ameliorate its effects on body function. A pathologist studies disease from the perspective of tissue and cell dysfunction. This term covers the study of everything from the appearance of dysfunctional cells to the gross appearance of diseased tissues and body malfunctions. If we trace what is or is not happening physiologically in an organ or system as opposed to starting from a structural abnormality, we are studying *pathophysiology*. *Histopathology* is the study of disease at the cellular or tissue level.

Do We Keep Track of Disease?

Epidemiologists are trained scientists who identify, study, and track disease in the populations of their individual areas. Although not all diseases are contagious, many diseases spread from smaller to larger populations of people or from animals to people or from insects to people. Epidemiologists are very important in formulating public health policy. Statistics related to the number of people in a given population who have a disease at a given time determine the *prevalence* of that disease. The number of new cases of a disease that appear in a population over a set period of time is known as the *incidence* rate. A high incidence of a particular disease indicates an *epidemic*. All physicians are aware of the list of U.S. reportable diseases, which are diseases a physician must report to the U.S. Public Health Service. *Mortality* indicates how many deaths result from particular disease exposure in a given population. Diseases may be classified as acute, sudden onset and of less than 3 months' duration, or slow onset but continuous duration. *Morbidity* describes the process of dying due to a specific disease. In public health terms, morbidity indicates how many people are afflicted with a specific disease state.

What Causes a Disease to Develop?

To study the *etiology* of a disease is to study the cause of a disease. Unfortunately, many diseases have no known cause and these diseases are referred to as *idiopathic* diseases. Of the disease causes that we know, many diseases derive from some sort of genetic mutation. These diseases are *heritable*. There are a group of diseases in which the body attacks itself. These are known as *autoimmune* diseases (see Chapter 6). A disease caused by an infectious or mobile agent such as a virus, bacteria, fungi, or other microorganism is an *infectious disease*. Diseases that are present at birth are called *congenital* diseases. In the study of diseases scientists have reported on the association of certain characteristics with the development of certain diseases. These are called risk factors because they presumably increase a person's probability of developing a specific disease. For example, excess body fat stores in a person with a family history of type 2 diabetes are a risk factor for that person with respect to developing diabetes. Another example is that smoking by an individual is a risk factor for developing lung cancer and other respiratory diseases. Last, age is a risk factor for a variety of degenerative diseases. As a person ages, there is an increased likelihood of developing diabetes, heart disease, senile dementia, and so forth. Risk factors are, in reality, statistical probabilities for the development of subsequent events. They are not causes and should not be assumed to be causal. They are merely statistical associations of characteristics with diseases. As an example, just because a person is old does not mean that the person is demented. Age is a risk factor for dementia but not the cause of the dementia. The same is true for elevated blood cholesterol levels. Although elevated blood cholesterol levels are a risk factor in coronary vessel disease, they may not cause the disease. There are some individuals with very high blood cholesterol levels who never develop coronary heart disease.

What Are Signs and Symptoms?

Every physiological state has its own set of characteristics. A disease state likewise has its characteristics. These are the signs and symptoms of that particular disease. The individual with these characteristics might complain of a certain type of pain in a specific area of the body or may indicate a rash or be found to have a fever. These are signs of disease. When further investigated, additional characteristics or symptoms might be observed. Depending on the initial observations, further examinations might be in order. A physician might order laboratory tests using blood and/or urine, and/or x-rays of a specific body part might be ordered. Depending on the results, additional, more sophisticated tests might be in order to help define the disease state presented in the patient. For example, an individual might complain of always being cold or always feeling tired. The physician might suspect anemia and order a blood test that will provide an estimation of number of red cells, hemoglobin content, and a differential red cell count. If the red cell count is below normal and there is a reduced hemoglobin content, the physician has substantiated his/her suspicions. The physician might then want to determine why the anemia developed and further tests might be ordered as well as an assessment of the patient's diet. If the diet is inadequate, the anemia might be a sign of malnutrition.

Diagnosis is the responsibility of the physician and associated healthcare providers. It is based on the examination of the patient and the results of a variety of tests. The physician then prescribes appropriate therapy for the condition presented. This might include specific medications, surgery, physical therapy, diet therapy, and other therapies designed to help the patient return to his/her normal homeostatic state.

What Kinds of Laboratory Work Could Be Helpful in Describing the Case?

For many situations very simple assessments are used. Measurements of the body weight and height, calculation of body mass index (weight/height^2), skin color and texture, ease of movement, and general appearance can be quite revealing. These observations can then be supported by assessments of key metabolites in blood and urine as well as levels of various components in the blood. Enzyme levels, for example, in blood can reveal tissue damage as occurs in a heart attack. Other enzyme levels can give information about how certain prescribed drugs are being tolerated by the body. In the preceding chapter are several tables illustrating the measurements that can be made in blood and urine that will provide information about the physiological state of the body. Deviations from normal can indicate or be characteristic of certain disease states.

What Kinds of Tissues Can Be Used for Laboratory Assessment?

For the simple, straightforward assessments of metabolism, blood and urine can be used. The values for many of these measurements from normal adult humans were shown in Chapter 1 (Tables 1.3, 1.4, and 1.5). Usually the individual is asked to fast prior to having a sample of blood drawn. This is to ensure that baseline measurements are made. Sometimes blood samples are drawn before and after the administration of a drug or a food or a specific nutrient to determine how well that item is handled by the body. Urine samples can be either randomly collected or collected over a specific period of time, for example, 24 hours.

If there is a need, biopsies of specific tissues can be made. A biopsy is a very small tissue sample. If from an easily accessed tissue such as skin or adipose or muscle, the site for biopsy is made numb and a tiny sample is taken. If a biopsy is needed from an organ such as the liver or kidney, more than site-specific numbness will be required. These deep biopsy samples are not drawn unless there is a really important reason for doing so and there are no other ways of getting the desired results to pinpoint a diagnosis.

Beyond these simple, easily accessed tissues that can be used for clinical analyses, there are more complicated tests that are used by the clinician and/or researcher. For example, if one wishes to know the density of the skeletal system in order to assess the presence of bone disease, the dual energy x-ray absorptiometry (DEXA) method is used. This is a sophisticated instrument that uses computers to measure bone density from x-rays and from information on the weight and height of the individual. This instrument can also compute or estimate the proportion of the body that is fat. The case studies presented in this book provide results of the simpler methods of assessments, and where complicated methods are used, an explanation is provided.

How Long Does a Disease Last?

The time course of each particular disease is sometimes difficult to predict. This is due in part to individual variability and on the type of disease. Sometimes the condition can be rapidly reversed with appropriate management; other times the condition is long lasting. For example, the duration of a common cold might be anywhere from 7 days to 2 weeks. The mending of a bone fracture in a young healthy individual might take 6 weeks, while in another older individual it might take much longer. Reversal of pyridoxine deficiency can take 6 minutes when pyridoxine is infused into the vein of the deficient child. Reversal of vitamin A deficiency might take several weeks, depending on the degree of malnutrition. Reversal of excess fat stores (obesity) might take a year of continual food intake restriction. So much depends on the type of disease, the individual afflicted, and the treatments available for its reversal. Primary to a successful outcome is the rapid and accurate assessment of the problem and the prompt administration of appropriate treatment. It must be noted, however, that not all diseases have appropriate and successful treatments. Sometimes a disease outbreak or epidemic occurs that suggests that there might be environmental factors at work. Under these circumstances, the U.S. Public Health Service, Centers for Disease Control (CDC) sends a team of investigators to find the reasons why the epidemic is occurring. This team gathers a variety of information about both the afflicted and those who are healthy in order to understand the nature of the problem. This is called an *epidemiological* approach to disease management. The following exercise will give you, the reader, an idea of how this might work.

Learning Activity 2.1: Epidemiology Case Study

The following case is adapted from information submitted to the CDC in Atlanta. Completing the parts of this case study will help you practice the use of case studies and help you to understand how diseases are followed across the country.

Suspected Legionnaires' Disease in Bogalusa*

The Story

On October 31, 1989, the state health department in Louisiana was notified by two physicians in Bogalusa that over 50 cases of acute pneumonia (severe infection of the lungs) had occurred among local residents. Most cases had occurred within a 3-week interval in mid- to late October; six persons had died. All cases had occurred in adults. The information the doctors had obtained from several patients suggested that the cause of the illness may have been legionellosis, a disease caused by infection with the bacterium *Legionella pneumophila*.

To answer the following questions, put yourself in the position of the EIS officer (a CDC disease detective) assigned to coordinate this study with that of the Louisiana Health Department. You have just received a telephone call from concerned physicians in Bogalusa, Louisiana. Ask yourself the following: Based on scientific method used by researchers, what additional information would help you decide whether this is potentially a real public health problem? (Hint: Look up Legionnaires' disease. Find out what causes it and what environmental circumstances stimulate its spread.)

Continue with this story only after you have answered the above question. Serologic testing is the analysis of samples of blood serum for the presence of antibodies to specific disease agents, including bacteria and viruses. Some antibodies indicate recent infection and are called IgM class; antibodies indicating more distant past infection are called IgG. In Bogalusa, blood samples obtained from several patients during the early (acute) phase of illness had been negative for antibody to the *Legionella* bacterium. (Note, however, that for most infectious diseases antibodies cannot be detected during the first few weeks in the course of illness.) No sputum specimens had been collected for Legionnaires' testing, since the hospital's laboratory was not able to perform the test on sputum. Now, ask yourself the next question: In general, besides *Legionella*, what could have accounted for the sudden increase in the number of cases of a pneumonia that had been reported to the Louisiana Health Department?

The story continues: The following information about Legionnaires' disease is abstracted from the publication *Control of Communicable Diseases Manual, 16th edition*. (In an actual epidemiological investigation, you might consult a reference publication such as this or a past textbook to refresh your memory on pertinent details about a specific disease.)

Now then, you have looked up Legionnaires' disease and have learned that this disease, or legionellosis, is characterized by pneumonia caused by the bacterium *Legionella pneumophila*. The name *Legionnaires' disease* was given to this problem following a large outbreak among persons who attended a convention of American Legion military veterans in Philadelphia, Pennsylvania, in July 1976. The incubation period (the amount of time from

---

* Adapted from http://www.cdc.gov/excite/PDF/LegionaQ.pdf accessed 10/2/08.

initial exposure to the infectious bacteria to the actual onset of illness) for Legionnaires' disease ranges from 2 to 10 days. The disease often begins with anorexia (loss of appetite), malaise (fatigue and overall sense of "feeling bad"), myalgias (muscle aches and soreness), and headache, followed by rapidly rising fever and chills. Chest x-rays typically show patchy areas of inflammation and fluid accumulation in the lungs. The diagnosis is confirmed by one of the following:

1. Isolation of the bacterium on special culture media
2. Demonstration of the bacterium by an immunofluorescent stain of involved tissue or respiratory secretions
3. A fourfold or greater increase in titers of antibodies to *L. pneumophila* in blood between the acute (early) illness and the convalescent period (long-term [usually 3 to 4 weeks] after the acute period)
4. A single high titer in a patient with an illness characterized by the symptoms and/or signs of Legionnaires' disease

Reading further, you learn that cases of Legionnaires' disease occur sporadically (individually) and in outbreaks. The reservoirs of the *L. pneumophila* bacteria responsible for many of these outbreaks have been primarily aqueous, and are found in such environments as hot water systems, air conditioning cooling towers, and evaporator condensers, all of which provide a moist environment conducive to the growth of this bacterium. The mode of transmission is airborne via aerosol-producing devices. Because *L. pneumophila* is spread by the airborne route from environmental sources (and not via person-to-person contact), when outbreaks are detected, there is a need for a speedy response. The common source in the environment must be identified and decontaminated to prevent the occurrence of additional cases. Risk factors for serious illness include increasing age, smoking, diabetes, chronic lung disease, renal (kidney) disease, cancer, and immune-compromised states. More men than women develop the disease. The ratio of men to women is 2.5:1.

Background on Bogalusa

Bogalusa is located in Washington Parish, Louisiana, and has a population of about 16,000. The largest employer is a paper mill located in the center of town adjacent to the main street. The paper mill includes five prominent industrial cooling towers. The mill also has three paper machines that emit large volumes of aerosol along the main street in town. Bogalusa is served by a 98-bed private hospital (hospital A) and a 60-bed public hospital (hospital B). Three additional hospitals are located in the surrounding parish. All of the reported cases of Legionnaires' disease were for patients at hospital A. The number of patients discharged with a diagnosis of pneumonia at hospital A since January 1986 is shown in Table 2.1. Between January 1986 and September 1989, only one pneumonia patient had been diagnosed as having Legionnaires' disease. A review of the charts of pneumonia patients at hospital A during October revealed that many patients were admitted with a febrile illness characterized by weakness, lethargy, and mental confusion. Some patients had a dry cough, and several reported having watery diarrhea. Chest x-rays were consistent with pneumonia. Most cases were residents of Bogalusa or the surrounding areas of Washington Parish.

Now answer the following question: What are the possible interpretations for the data in the table below? (It may help to restructure the data into a bar graph.) Develop some hypotheses about why Bogalusa residents are getting sick.

Table 2.1 Number of Patients with a Diagnosis of Pneumonia
Discharged from Hospital A by Month, 1986–1989

	1986	1987	1988	1989
January	12	20	21	16
February	14	19	26	19
March	7	21	8	27
April	12	10	11	13
June	4	11	1	6
July	5	5	9	8
August	5	9	12	7
September	6	7	13	8
October	15	8	10	70
November	?	8	10	
December		11	20	
Total	75	129	153	174

Continuing the story: Discussions were held among staff of the Louisiana Health Department and the CDC. The health department felt capable of leading the epidemiological investigation, but requested assistance with laboratory support. A second EIS officer was sent from Atlanta to assist in the investigation, and CDC provided laboratory support. The field investigation team arrived in Bogalusa in early November.

The EIS officers were given the opportunity to address the hospital staff about this outbreak. In addition to being certain that hospital staff could recognize (diagnose) and appropriately treat patients with Legionnaires' disease, the investigators needed to enlist the hospital staff to provide their cooperation and assistance with the investigation. Some of the points they covered during the meeting were:

- The clinical features of Legionnaires' disease, methods for diagnosis, and the specimens that will be needed for laboratory analysis
- The basic epidemiological features of Legionnaires' disease including risk for disease and sources for infection
- Why it is important to report cases promptly and how to report to public health authorities
- How to treat the infection (the antibiotic erythromycin was recommended)
- What is known to date regarding the outbreak
- Plans for the continuing epidemiological investigation

The investigators set up an active surveillance protocol that included the collection, analysis, and dissemination of data on illness and the means for finding cases at all five hospitals in the Bogalusa area. In addition, they used a questionnaire to acquire information from the medical records of all persons admitted or discharged with a diagnosis of pneumonia, respiratory distress, or possible Legionnaires' disease since October 1, 1989.

A possible case of Legionnaires' disease was defined as an illness in a resident or visitor of Washington Parish (where Bogalusa is located), who was greater than 20 years of age. This individual was admitted to one of the hospitals after October 1, 1989, with x-ray evidence of pneumonia or a chest radiograph consistent with pneumonia. A confirmed case had to meet the criteria for a possible case, plus have lab evidence of Legionnaires' disease (fourfold rise in antibody titer, a single elevated convalescent antibody titer, positive urine antigen test, positive sputum culture, or positive biopsy).

By November 19, investigators had identified 83 patients who met the definition of possible Legionnaires' disease. Fourteen of these patients died before *Legionella* testing could be performed. Of the 83, 65% were female. About three-quarters of the case-patients were residents of Bogalusa; about one-half (41) resided on the east side of town. Most case-patients had been admitted to the hospital in mid-October; few if any new cases occurred in mid-November. To date, no sputum culture had shown growth for Legionnaires' disease or other pathogens.

Based on the hypotheses you developed for the preceding question, what would be your strategy for proving or disproving your ideas about how the people of Bogalusa are getting sick? How would you summarize your data related to the frequency of pneumonia in Bogalusa?

Conclusion

As you think about this case and develop your responses to the questions posed above, you will find that you have learned a lot about lung function, pneumonia, differential diagnosis, population studies, and strategies for identifying and eliminating the described problem. In this instance, there might not be any nutritional implications, *or* are there? Could you think about whether nutritional status had anything to do with the susceptibility of people to this disease? You should look at sources of information about immunity and nutrition. There might be some relationship. Make a list of the associations you find from your library research into this topic.

chapter 3

Homeostasis

What Is Homeostasis?

Homeostasis (homeo = same, stasis = stay) is a term used to describe the condition of balance of the internal environment in the body where a variety of regulatory processes work to maintain constancy of these internal systems within operational limits. The regulation of body temperature and pH are two examples of homeostatic regulation. Other examples include the body's relatively stable blood glucose and electrolyte concentrations and acid-base balance. Much of this regulation occurs via a system of communication orchestrated by the endocrine system. This system releases hormones in response to both external and internal signals. The hormones in turn travel in the blood from their point of origin to their target tissues, which in turn respond to this shift in the environment. This can be visualized as a cascade: A change in the environment leads to a hormone response that in turn leads to a metabolic response. In many cases the brain is the master orchestrator of this response. As discussed in Chapter 2, when homeostasis is perturbed and not re-established, disease can result. Sometimes when homeostasis is perturbed, the body adjusts to this perturbation and a new homeostatic regulatory state is achieved. This is called *adaptation*. An example of this is when an individual leaves a warm environment and enters a cold environment. Perhaps the individual lives in Florida and has taken a trip to Vermont in February. This individual has managed to thrive in Florida's warm and humid environment. Now, having flown to Vermont where it is drier and much colder, with ice and snow, this individual will need to adjust to this change in environmental conditions. At first with a light coat on, the individual feels cold. Shivering occurs and the individual generates additional body heat via brown fat thermogenesis. The individual also modifies his/her behavior: puts on a warm coat, hat, gloves, and boots. Upon arrival, he/she minimizes time spent out of doors in the cold and enters a heated building. Since this individual has come to Vermont to ski, of course staying indoors is not an option. The next day, skiing commences. So, what has happened? He/she has adjusted to the temperature change. With adjustment (adaptation), shivering and brown fat thermogenesis declined and the vacation begins. The individual has set a new homeostatic level so that he/she can survive the cold conditions of Vermont. When he/she returns to Florida, the adaptation to the environment in Florida will reverse the adaptation to Vermont. These kinds of adaptations occur throughout life. Usually they are not noticed except if the individual happens to recall an event such as this trip to a cold environment or conversely a trip to a hot one. Setting a new homeostatic level is often an unconscious event.

How Is Homeostasis Regulated?

Signals to and from the brain may be part of the response to a change in the environment. For example, you might be taking a stroll in the country when, much to your dismay, a galloping bull is spotted heading straight toward you. You become alarmed and run toward a fence and jump over it. The external environment changed (the appearance of the bull) and your internal environment changed in response (your fight-or-flight response kicked in). You perceived the danger, ran faster than you ever thought you could, and jumped higher than you had ever jumped before. Signals to the heart and to the lungs were a part of this response. The heart rate increased, the muscles contracted and relaxed working hard to allow you to run away, your respiratory rate increased to provide more oxygen to the red blood cells for delivery to the working muscles, and blood flowed faster to and from the periphery. All of these responses were coordinated by a very efficient signaling system involving the release of hormones that in turn were bound to structures called *receptors* in or on the cells of the target tissues. When bound, these hormones elicited a response appropriate to the change in the environment. After you had escaped the dangerous bull and were safely on the other side of the fence, your body then returned to its prior relaxed state, but it took some time. Your brain perceived that you were out of danger. Neurotransmitters were released that counteracted the neurotransmitters that were released as part of the fight-or-flight response, and your heart rate slowed down, as did your respiratory rate. Your muscles relaxed and homeostasis was again restored. Note how many systems were involved: your neuronal system, your musculoskeletal system, your respiratory system, your vascular system, and of course, your endocrine system. This signaling system (signals as well as the receptors on the target tissues) is designed to maintain life in as normal a condition as possible.

The receptors are sometimes referred to as effectors because they carry out the response elicited by the signal whether it is a hormone or a metabolite or an ion. Effectors are cell structures, usually proteins, that bind the hormone(s) sent by the control center. Through binding, a response is implemented that allows the body to regulate its activity within the framework of homeostasis. Changes to variables and the re-establishment of homeostasis is a normal and on-going process. Thus, homeostasis is not a static, one-time event but is instead a dynamic and ongoing one.

As mentioned above and in Chapter 2, should homeostasis be perturbed and the individual is unable to return to the prior state of healthy homeostasis, then health consequences may follow. Again, using the above example of the stroll in the country and the charging bull, suppose the individual was a 70-year-old man with high blood pressure (hypertension) and arthritis. He spots the bull and his fight-or-flight response kicks in. However, although he might be swift enough to escape and is not mauled by the bull, his fight-or-flight response (a large sudden increase in the neurotransmitter epinephrine) elevates his blood pressure. This is a sudden rise that is part of the fight-or-flight response. However, this 70-year-old man has a vascular system that has lost some of its elasticity (hence his hypertension). As a consequence, this man is unable to dilate one or more of the blood vessels in his brain, and due to the increase in pressure the blood vessel bursts and he has a stroke. His body was unable to swiftly and *correctly* counteract the neurotransmitters of the flight-or-fight response. His heart rate and blood pressure rose, but his aging vascular system could not expand sufficiently to allow the increased blood flow to and from his vital organs and to and from his periphery. Here is an example of a disease state (stroke preceded by the hypertension due to the loss in elasticity of the vascular system) that is a perturbation of homeostasis. There was a failure to return to the prior state of relaxation because with age there was a change in the internal environment that compromised the cascade of responses to the change in the external environment.

Species differ in how they regulate their body systems to maintain homeostasis. For example, humans regulate their body temperature by sweating in a hot environment. Dogs do not sweat but instead pant to rid their body of excess heat. Both processes are homeostatic mechanisms for maintaining body temperature at that species's ideal temperature.

Species differ in their optimal body temperature. Chickens, for example, have a body temperature that is 4 degrees higher than the human's body temperature of 98.4°F.

Oxygen consumption and carbon dioxide release is another system that is homeostatically regulated. Sometimes it is connected to body temperature regulation. Consider a bear that is in hibernation. When hibernating, it is in a semiconscious state. It is deeply asleep. It uses very little oxygen and its body temperature is lowered. The bear is in a state of suspended animation. Another example is fish. They acquire their oxygen by swimming through the water. Water passes over their gills and the oxygen that is dissolved in the water is extracted. Some fish are very active swimmers; others are not. Those that are not acquire (and need) much less oxygen than their active counterparts. The homeostatic mechanism for the "lazy" fish is a bit different from the active fish. The lazy fish needs less oxygen and is more likely closer to a state of suspended animation than is the active fish. Should the water be depleted of oxygen, as happens with an overgrowth of algae (an algae bloom), the fish will die.

What Is the Relevance of Homeostatic Control to Our Understanding of the Physiology of Nutrition?

Homeostasis is maintained through a whole system of checks and balances that ensure survival of the species. However, in some cases, attempts to regain homeostasis fail and disease results. As an example, some people may consciously try to control their food intake to the extreme. People can become obsessed with the desire to be thin and either refuse to eat and adequately nourish their bodies or eat and then force themselves to regurgitate the food. Self-induced vomiting is called *bulimia* or *bulimia nervosa*. Additional behavior related to an obsession with body weight includes the excessive use of laxatives and diuretics and the extensive participation in exercise designed to increase energy expenditure. Although the patients may be eating some food, they are not consuming enough food to meet their macro- and micronutrient requirements. This is known as *anorexia* or *anorexia nervosa*. Because of these behaviors, they are in negative energy and protein balance; that is, they are not consuming enough energy-rich and protein-rich foods to meet their energy and protein need. They are malnourished. These patients are characterized by little body fat. The normal body contains 10–20% fat; the anorexic body may contain less than 5%. Amenorrhea (in females), hypothermia (feeling cold and unable to generate sufficient body heat to feel warm), and hypotension (low blood pressure) can develop. If the excessive weight loss is unrecognized and untreated, anorexics may starve to death. Some people, for whatever reason, self-recognize and resume eating.

In many respects, anorexic people have physiological/biochemical features that are similar to those patients who are starved. Their catabolic hormone levels are high and their body-energy stores are being raided as a result. Insulin resistance due to the catabolic hormones is observed. Liver and muscle glycogen levels are low. Fat stores are minimal. As the weight loss proceeds further, these individuals have reduced bone mass, decreased metabolic rate, decreased heart rate, hypoglycemia, hypothyroidism, electrolyte imbalance, elevated free fatty acid and cholesterol levels, peripheral edema, and finally cardiac and renal failure. When their fat stores fall below 2% of total body weight, they will die. This 2% represents the lipids essential to the structure and function of membranes as well as those complex lipids that are components of the central nervous system. With this scenario in mind, the clinician faces the challenge of reversing the condition. Just as it is difficult to reverse starvation-induced changes in the metabolism of unintentionally starving humans, reversing the weight loss of anorexic patients presents some special challenges. The energy requirements for weight regain in anorexic patients are highly variable and depend largely on the physiological status of the patient at the time of treatment initiation and on the pre-anorexia body weight. Those patients who had been obese prior to their self-induced anorexia regained their lost weight faster than patients who had been of normal body weight. Successful treatment of anorexia nervosa is associated with increases in bone mineral density as well as improvement in other measures of body composition. The outcome of the treatment depends on the time at which it is instituted. If anorexia nervosa is recognized early in the sequence of hormonal and metabolic change, then the chances of success are much greater than if treatment is initiated after irreversible tissue changes have occurred. While controversy exists as to the success of treatment as well as the accuracy of diagnosis, it is generally agreed that aggressive treatment can achieve reversal in 50% of the cases. Mortality is estimated in 6% of cases. This leaves an estimate of approximately 44% who recover spontaneously without medical intervention. Included in the mortality figure of 6% are those who commit suicide. This implies a relationship between the development of depression and anorexia—two self-destructive behaviors that represent abnormalities in the central nervous system (CNS).

Bulimic and nonbulimic anorexics differ in their weight recovery. Those who were bulimic recover their lost weight more rapidly than those who were anorexic only. This is probably due to the difference in rate of weight loss. Those anorexics who were also bulimic were more severely starved and lost weight faster than nonbulimic anorexics. Because of this, bulimics are more likely to be diagnosed and treated sooner than nonbulimic anorexics. In anorexics, as with prolonged starvation, gut absorptive capacity is compromised due to a loss of cells lining the gastrointestinal tract. In the early phase of treatment, malabsorption is likely to occur. For this reason, the diet offered during recovery must be gradually increased with respect to its energy content. This also applies to a person who has been starving. A gradual 300 kcal thrice weekly increase from an initial 1200 kcal diet that includes about 3g sodium is recommended. The recovery diet should also be a lactose-free diet and should be offered in six or more small meals over 24 hours. A low-fat diet is sometimes recommended, but this depends on the genetic background and pre-anorexia or prestarvation health status of the patient. Those with diabetic tendencies might not fare as well if faced with a low-fat–high-carbohydrate diet. The medical history of the patient and family will provide clues as to the most appropriate diet design. The recovering anorexic requires more food than the recovering bulimic anorexic. The recovering anorexic has lost more absorptive cells than the bulimic anorexic. Of interest is the report that even after weight regain, the recovered anorexic has a higher than normal energy requirement and, if this is not met, will begin to lose weight once again. This suggests that not all anorexia nervosa is self-inflicted. It may begin with a conscious effort to consume less food but then may continue because of a change in the signals for food-intake initiation and cessation and a change in the efficiency with which the body uses the food consumed.

Malnutrition as Part of a Homeostatic Disturbance

Starvation is the extreme state of malnutrition that occurs when the individual is provided little or no food to nourish the body. Between starvation and the state of adequate nourishment to meet nutrient needs, there are graded levels of inadequate nutrient intake. Although infants and children of third-world nations come to mind when malnutrition is pictured, people of all ages in all countries are vulnerable. Where the intake of macro-nutrients is inadequate, the syndrome is called *protein-calorie malnutrition* (PCM) or, more correctly, *protein-energy malnutrition*.

Chronic malnutrition is characterized not only by energy deficit (energy need exceeding energy intake) but also by a deficit in the protein intake and the intake of micronutrients. The needs for these nutrients and energy are determined by the age and health status of the individual being assessed. Examples of factors contributing to malnutrition include rapid growth, infection, injury, poor health practices, and chronic debilitating disease. Each of these conditions can increase the demand for the nutrients in food. For example, excessive use of laxatives over a long period of time can result in PCM because the use of laxatives reduces the availability of essential nutrients to the body. Where food is in short supply, growing children are likely to develop PCM. Patients in hospitals who cannot or will not consume adequate amounts of food are at risk for malnutrition.

Poorly nourished individuals not only lose their energy reserves but also have distur-bances in their electrolyte balance. The electrolytes of concern are sodium, potassium, cal-cium, phosphorus, and magnesium. Disturbances in either the intake or the conservation of these electrolytes by the body can have serious consequences.

Sodium

Sodium (Na^+) is the major extracellular electrolyte. It has an important role in muscle func-tion. When muscles contract they do so via a mechanism that uses the exchange of sodium for potassium. The muscle then relaxes and the shift is reversed. This shift uses a mecha-nism called the *sodium-potassium ATPase* and another system called the *sodium-calcium anti-port system*. Calcium triggers muscle contraction, which, as mentioned, involves the inflow of sodium. As muscles contract and relax, these electrolytes move back and forth between the extracellular and intracellular compartments.

It has been estimated that the adult body contains 52–60 mEq of sodium/kg (male) and 48–55 mEq/kg (female). One meq/L equals one mmol/L. The average adult male has about 83–97 g of sodium in his 70 kg body. Between 2/3 and 3/4 of this sodium is "fixed" in the mineral apatite of the bone. The remainder enters a pool that undergoes consider-able flux as it participates in sodium–potassium exchange. The serum contains 136–145 mEq/L of sodium. Normal sodium intake varies from less than 2 grams to 10 grams per day. Most of this sodium comes from table salt, NaCl. Foods rich in added salt are usually snack foods such as potato chips, salted nuts, and pretzels. Every living thing and the food that nourishes it contains sodium and, except for pure fats and carbohydrates, no major food source lacks this element. Heavy work in a hot, dry environment and a variety of medical conditions will affect the need for sodium as well as for other electrolytes that are lost through the skin. While sodium intake can be highly variable, serum sodium is not. As described above, the normal range of serum sodium is quite small. Serum values in excess of 150 mEq/L (hypernatremia) are considered abnormal. Values below 135 mEq/L (hyponatremia) are also considered abnormal and are of clinical concern. In normal indi-viduals the level of sodium in the serum is tightly controlled and this control is inter-twined with the control of potassium concentration, chloride concentration, and water balance. Diarrhea, due to illness or to the excessive use of laxatives, increases the loss of both sodium and potassium. Excessive sweating over a period of time likewise can result in an excessive loss of these electrolytes.

Potassium

Potassium (K^+) is the major intracellular electrolyte. The healthy young adult male has between 42 and 48 mEq K^+/kg body weight or 2940–3360 mEq in the 70 kg man. Persons with above-average muscle mass, for example, athletes, will have more body potassium than persons of average muscle mass. Virtually all the body potassium is exchangeable, with the exception of small amounts that are irretrievably bound up in the bone mineral. The Na^+K^+ATPase actively works to ensure that K^+ stays within the cell and that very little (3.5–5.0 mEq/L) is present in extracellular fluids.

Just as all foods serve as sources of sodium, so too are they sources of potassium. Only highly refined food ingredients, for example, pure sugars, fats, and oils, lack this essential nutrient. Especially good sources are orange juice, avocados, fish, and bananas. Potassium passes freely from the gastrointestinal system into the enterocytes lining the intestinal tract and then into the body. Potassium is distributed in response to energy-dependent Na^+ redistribution. Almost all of the consumed potassium in excess of need is excreted in the urine, with a very small amount found in the feces in healthy, normal adults. In persons experiencing diarrhea, however, the loss of potassium can be quite large and debilitating. If the diarrhea is of short duration (less than 12 hours) the body will compensate and the person will survive. However, should this condition persist, potassium supplementation will be needed. Such is the case for a number of malabsorption syndromes. The plasma or serum level of potassium is not a reliable index of whole-body potassium status simply because potassium within the cell (not the serum) is the critical value rather than the more measurable serum values. Causes for concern with too little potassium (hypokalemia) or too much (hyperkalemia) have to do with muscle contractility. If hypokalemia persists, the person could die of cardiac arrest. This occurs because too much K^+ has left the contractile unit and the heart muscle loses its ability to contract. The regulation of potassium balance follows that of sodium.

Chloride

Chloride (Cl^-) likewise is related to sodium and potassium balance. As an electronegative element, chloride is a good oxidizing agent. One of its main functions is as an essential ingredient of the gastric acid, hydrochloric acid. The gastric juice contains 120–160 mEq of chloride/L. Another major function of chloride aside from its passive participation in electrolyte balance has to do with hemoglobin and its function as a carrier of oxygen and carbon dioxide. The process is called the *chloride shift*. It works by using the chloride ion as a modulator of hemoglobin oxygen binding affinity. The Cl^- is bound more tightly to deoxyhemoglobin than to oxyhemoglobin. Hence, the affinity of hemoglobin is directly proportional to the concentration of Cl^-. The carbonate ion HCO_3^- freely permeates the erythrocyte membrane so that once formed, it equilibrates with the plasma. The need for charge neutrality on both sides of the red cell membrane requires that Cl^- replace HCO_3^- as it leaves the erythrocyte. Consequently, because cations do not shift, the Cl^- ion in the venous blood erythrocyte is higher than in the arterial blood erythrocyte. Thus the Cl^- modulates hemoglobin oxygen affinity.

Normal chloride levels in plasma are 100–106 mEq/L and vary very little. The glomerular filtrate contains 108 mEq/L and urine contains 138 mEq/L. Sweat can contain as much as 40 mEq/L but usually contains only trace amounts. The intracellular fluid contains very little Cl^- (~4 mEq/L), whereas intestinal juice contains 69–127 mEq/L. In instances of secretory diarrhea, the chloride content of the excrement can be as high as 45 mEq/L.

Most of the chloride in the intestinal tract does not appear in the feces of normal individuals. Rather, this ion recirculates as sodium and potassium are carried into the body. The main excretory pathway is urine. This ion is passively distributed throughout the body. As described above, it moves to replace anions lost to cells via other processes. It is the other half of table salt, NaCl, and as such, is found in abundance in most foods. Dietary intake is in excess of that of sodium, yet the usual plasma $Na^+:Cl^-$ ratio is about 3:2. This imbalance is due to the passive nature of chloride transfer between water compartments and to the active system that serves to retain Na^+. Instances of below and above normal plasma levels of Cl^- are not diet related but are due to metabolic reasons usually related to the regulation of Na^+ and K^+ homeostasis.

Calcium

Calcium (Ca^{++}) is the primary mineral in bones and teeth, where it is present as hydroxyapatite ($3Ca_3(PO_4)_2 \bullet Ca(OH)_2$). On a dry-weight basis, bone contains about 150 mg calcium/gram bone. By comparison, soft tissue such as liver, muscle, or brain contains less than 35 µg calcium/gram tissue. A normal 70 kg man will have about 22 mg calcium/gram fat-free tissue or a total of 1.54 kg calcium. While the calcium in the teeth is seldom mobilized, that which is in the skeletal muscle is mobilized and replaced at about 0.5 g/day. This daily turnover of calcium is essential to the maintenance of metabolic homeostasis because not only does calcium serve as a structural element, in its ionized form, it also serves as an essential element in cell signaling systems. Of the total body calcium, 1% serves as an intracellular/intercellular messenger/regulator. Calcium mobilization and deposition changes with age, diet, hormonal status, and physiological state. Bone calcium homeostasis is related to bone strength and if mobilization exceeds deposition, the bones will become porous (osteoporosis). The very compact cortical portions of the bone disappear, leaving a fragile, largely trabecular bone. The result of these changes is a fragile skeletal system that breaks easily. Inadequate calcium intakes as well as inadequate phosphorus and magnesium intakes can lead to inadequate bone mineralization (osteomalacia).

The muscle cell has a unique calcium storage site in the sarcoplasmic reticulum. This reticulum is similar to that found in other cell types but is highly specialized. It contains large quantities of calcium-activated ATPase. Approximately 75% of the sarcoplasmic reticulum is this ATPase. The ATPase also requires magnesium, so its name indicates this: $Ca^{++}Mg^{++}ATPase$. It serves as a calcium pump using the energy released by ATP to drive the calcium ion from the cytosol to the sarcoplasmic reticulum. There the calcium resides until needed for muscle contraction. Upon receipt of a signal to contract, a Ca^{++} channel is opened and Ca^{++} flows into the cytoplasm of the muscle cell whereupon it binds to troponin, a contractile protein of skeletal and cardiac muscle. When Ca^{++} binds to it, the troponin changes its shape, becoming shorter. The muscle cell contains two other filaments, actin and myosin, which interact when troponin shortens due to Ca^{++} binding. When troponin is in the relaxed state these two filaments are too far apart to interact.

Muscles are signaled to contract by a wave of depolarization–repolarization flowing down the muscle fiber from its point of contact at the neuromuscular junction. During depolarization of skeletal muscle, extracellular Na^+ flows into the cell and potentiates the Ca^{++} release from the sarcoplasmic reticulum. In the heart muscle, with its slightly different muscle fiber organization, the signal for contraction is generated by the AV sinus node on the right side of the heart. This signal is regularly spaced and results in depolarization–repolarization just as happens in skeletal muscle. However, with depolarization, Ca^{++} flows into the cytosol from the extracellular fluid as well as from the sarcoplasmic reticulum. This has the result of increasing the strength of the contraction because more calcium is present. During repolarization Ca^{++} is then pumped, via the Ca^{++} Mg^{++} pump, back into the sarcoplasmic reticulum. In heart muscle there are many more mitochondria providing ATP than are found in skeletal muscle; hence the need for Ca^{++} by the heart muscle is greater than that by skeletal muscle.

Magnesium

Magnesium (Mg^{++}) is another of the important electrolytes for muscle contraction. Magnesium deficiency is characterized by very low blood levels of magnesium and neuromuscular symptoms such as muscle spasms, twitching, muscle fasciculations, tremor, personality changes, anorexia, nausea, and vomiting. Marginally deficient states have been suggested in patients with normal serum or blood levels but depleted tissue levels of magnesium. In these patients the symptoms are varied and it may be difficult to assign magnesium deficiency as their cause unless tissue samples (muscle) are obtained and assayed. A positive magnesium balance of 1 mEq/kg can be demonstrated in such individuals. Frequently, magnesium deficiency is accompanied by hypocalcemia. This is due to a failure of bone to exchange calcium for magnesium.

Other Instances of Homeostatic Regulation

Growth and Development

Homeostasis is also at work in growth. From the single fertilized cell to maturity, the human passes through several important stages: conception to birth, infanthood, childhood, adolescence, and finally adulthood. Each of the growth stages is characterized by both an increase in cell number and a concerted and coordinated change in cell/tissue/organ characteristics and function. Longitudinal growth of the skeleton is the most obvious feature, accompanied by the growth and maturation of the muscles, the internal organs, the reproductive system, and the central nervous system. Physical activity and the consumption of a well-balanced diet adequate in all the needed nutrients ensure this coordinated growth pattern. Should one or more of the essential nutrients be inadequate, growth abnormalities will be observed. Chronic laxative use, especially by a person who is growing rapidly, may disturb gastrointestinal function and promote diarrhea. In turn, this will reduce gut passage time and thus absorptive cell exposure time for nutrients. This perturbation in homeostasis results in malnutrition. The presence of intestinal parasites can also decrease nutrient availability to the host. Malnutrition will result here as well.

Obesity

Obesity is a form of malnutrition that occurs when homeostasis is perturbed by the ingestion of far more food energy than is needed to sustain the body and support its functions. Excess food intake is called *hyperphagia*. When this occurs, excess fat stores result. A small excess results in an overweight person. A large excess results in obesity. There are variations in the size of the fat stores that determine whether the person is thin, of normal weight for height and age, or is overweight or obese. Excess body-fat stores are considered a risk factor in a number of diseases and may be the result of an interaction between genetics and environment. An individual may have inherited one or more mutated genes that are associated with excess body fat stores. When provided with an ample food supply, these individuals may become fat. However, if the food supply is limited, the excess fat store might not develop. In addition, there may be cultural overrides that influence the phenotypic expression of an individual genotype. Individuals may consciously limit food intake and increase physical activity so as not to phenotypically express their genotype.

Food intake in excess of need (hyperphagia) may characterize the genetically obese human, yet there are many overfat people who are not hyperphagic. There are those who cannot dissipate their surplus intake energy as heat—that is, thermogenesis—and who do not tolerate cold well. It has been suggested that some genetically obese individuals become obese because they are unable to increase their heat production when overfed or when suddenly thrust into a cold environment.

Hyperphagia could also be due to a mutation in one of several of the hormones or their receptors that function in the regulation of food intake. The perceptions of hunger and satiety are the result of an interplay between these hormones and their receptors on the target tissues. Several individuals have been reported who do not produce normal leptin, a cytokine that works to suppress feeding when the fat stores are full. Leptin also stimulates heat production and helps the body keep warm under adverse conditions. Some individuals have normal leptin production but are abnormal with respect to the function of leptin because the cell structures that bind leptin are abnormal. This is a leptin receptor defect. The clinical characteristics are the same as in the person who does not produce useful leptin. Excess fat stores, hyperphagia, and reduced ability to respond to a cold environment are observed in these people. Normal-weight humans appear to regulate their body-fat mass by increasing their heat production when overfed or exposed to cold. As mentioned in the sections on starvation and anorexia, hormonal balance is important to the regulation of energy balance and normal body weight. Hypercortisolism and hyperinsulinism are associated with obesity. Cortisol and its related compounds, corticosterone and cortisone, play an important role in the regulation of fat synthesis and storage as well as in the signaling of apoptosis (programmed cell death). While these hormones are usually catabolic hormones, there are circumstances when they stimulate anabolic processes, such as fat synthesis.

Finally, there are social and cultural influences that can ensure or potentiate genetic tendencies to develop obesity. Anthropologists and medical historians have identified examples of cultural groups that consider excess body fat a mark of beauty as well as an indication of economic status within their society. Examples of this are the various statuary of the different ages all the way from the upper Paleolithic period through the Renaissance and the portraiture of wealthy individuals of the 18th and 19th centuries. Women have been represented with large bellies and breasts that, to the eye of the contemporary observer, are overfat. Men, too, are of ample proportions. In some cultures, female fatness may not only be a testament to the family's wealth, but also be a symbol of maternity and nurturance. This might be important to a woman in this culture if the only way she gains status is through motherhood. A fat woman was assumed to be very maternal and nurturing.

With respect to societal-determined fatness and the values of fatness, it can be assumed that the fatter a person is in a society that values fatness, the more likely that person will be to marry and produce children carrying genetic tendencies to be fat and who will be similarly taught to eat enough to be fat. Lean people will be less likely to contribute to the gene pool because they will be considered less-desirable mates. While people in the United States, as well as other developed nations, may not have these social values, there is no doubt that eating behaviors can be taught. If young children are constantly reminded and coached to overeat, there may be a continuing stimulus to over-consume food. Added to this

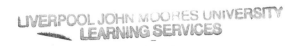

may be negative cultural and social dictates with respect to physical activity. A decrease in physical activity and energy expenditure ensures a positive energy balance that may well result in excess body fatness. The way to reduce the excess fat store not only involves eating less food so as to create an energy deficit but also to increase energy expenditure. By increasing energy expenditure (increasing physical activity) one can build muscle mass. Muscle burns more energy than adipose tissue. If one were to increase the muscle mass and reduce the fat mass, one would then increase basal energy expenditure. Basal energy expenditure (BMR, basal metabolic rate) is the amount of energy needed to sustain the body without any increments in energy to support physical activity. The effects of weight cycling (reducing one's food intake with consequent weight loss followed by resumption of food intake patterns and subsequent weight regain) on energy efficiency may be due to the composition of the weight loss during food restriction. One of the consequences of rapid weight loss, especially when induced by very low-energy, low-carbohydrate diets, is the loss of body protein or lean body mass. This is especially true when the individuals are physically inactive. Maintenance of lean body mass is an energy-expensive process. Lean body mass is the most metabolically active tissue in the body with respect to energy demands, accounting for the majority of the energy to support the basal energy requirement (i.e., 60–70% of daily basal energy requirements for adults). Therefore the less body protein, the lower the energy requirement. If weight loss consists of significant amounts of body protein, then the formerly overfat person will have a lower basal energetic requirement and an increased energy efficiency in terms of the weight regain as fat.

Homeostasis in Body Weight Regulation

Healthy adult humans vary very little over the years in their body weight. They may be overweight and/or overfat, but for most humans that weight is maintained for years until some event occurs that results in a body weight change. This is called the set-point theory. In women, pregnancy or menopause, two normal physiological events, may perturb homeostasis sufficiently to establish a new steady-state body weight (or new set point) that, again, will be tenaciously defended. A change in the endocrine system, an insult to the body, and a conscious decision to eat more (or less) over a prolonged period (months to years) are other examples of events that perturb homeostasis sufficiently to result in a new set point—a new body weight that is maintained from that time on.

Treatment of Obesity

In almost no other area of medicine have there been so many failures as have occurred in the treatment of obesity. The most common treatment is the reduction of food intake, which presumably means a reduction of energy intake.

Food restriction puts into place a metabolic machinery geared to save as much energy as possible and to stimulate the brain to signal the body to consume energy-rich foods. Thus, even though the patient tries to control eating and food intake, the body seeks to return to its prior overfat state. Constant vigilance is required of the patient to override these biological signals that direct the body to be fat. However, even when the patient carefully monitors food-energy intake and consciously decides to regulate it, weight regain may occur due to the body's increased energetic efficiency and its tendency to synthesize and store fat in preference to protein. This physiological defense may be counteracted by an increase in physical activity. Exercise, on a regular basis, stimulates muscle protein development and increases energy expenditure. Exercise can be a useful adjunct to energy-intake restriction because it redirects energy loss from the lean body mass to the adipose tissue fat stores. In the sedentary individual, weight loss occurs at the expense of both fat and protein components of the body. In the exercising food-restricted individual, the weight loss is primarily fat loss because the exercising muscles require a constant energy supply for their activity. This energy supply comes from the fat store. Further, mild to moderate exercise seems to suppress food intake. Thus, food restriction together with exercise is additive in a beneficial way with respect to the loss and regain of body fat. If the person is to maintain their newly acquired body weight, he/she must continue to exercise and monitor food intake. They cannot return to their prior sedentary overeating lifestyle.

Drugs in the Treatment of Obesity

Pharmacological approaches to the treatment of obesity have captured the interest of numerous pharmaceutical companies worldwide. Drugs that target mechanisms involved in hunger and satiety as well as drugs that target energy efficiency have been developed. The latter category includes compounds that interfere with normal digestion and absorption. Unfortunately, none of these compounds has a significant anti-obesity effect. Glucosidase inhibitors as well as lipase inhibitors have been developed. The glucosidase inhibitors, acarbose and miglitol, for example, inhibit the action of amylase and thus reduce its activity. This means that the long-chain (straight and branched) starches found in many plant products are not digested as quickly as usual. In theory, this retardation of digestion should result in a retardation of absorption of the end products of starch hydrolysis. Unfortunately, this may not result in a reduction in intake energy. If starch digestion is not completed by the enzymes of the small intestine, flora of the large intestine take over and produce fatty acids that are then absorbed and used for energy.

Lipase inhibitors (Xenecal or Orlistat) or fat absorption inhibitors (cholestyramine, neomycin, perflurooctyl bromide) also serve to reduce energy intake. Cholestyramine binds bile acids and disrupts micelle formation. This results in an inhibition of fat absorption and increased fecal fat loss. An over-the-counter drug, Alli, has recently been released. This is a weight loss drug sold in a lower dose than its parent drug, Orlestat. It was originally approved in 1999 as Xenical. The drug interferes with fat absorption and can help with weight loss if used as part of an overall weight loss program that includes exercise and the use of a low-fat diet. Because it inhibits fat absorption, very uncomfortable side effects are experienced if the food plan is not low fat. Gastrointestinal discomfort (bloating, gas, loose to runny stools) occurs in varying degrees.

Diet Products

Food companies have expanded into the "anti-obesity business" by developing noncaloric sweeteners, reduced-caloric sweeteners, fat substitutes, and bulking agents. All of these products are designed to reduce the energy value of food products. Aspartame, cyclamate, saccharin, and acesulfame K, and a mixture of dextrose, maltodextrin, and sucralose (Splenda) are sweeteners without energy value. Theoretically, aspartame could have an energy value since it is a dipeptide of phenylalanine and aspartic acid, but because it is 180 times sweeter than sucrose and is unstable in water and to heat, it is unlikely that significant amounts of this product will be consumed. So, for practical purposes, this sweetener would not contribute energy in any significant amount to the daily intake. Noncaloric sweeteners are used in soft drinks as well as in a number of snack foods. Canned fruit and frozen desserts are also prepared with these noncaloric sweeteners. Some of the sugar alcohols—for example, mannitol—are also used in prepared foods to reduce their energy content. Likewise, fat substitutes such as the sucrose polyester Olestra are used to reduce the energy value of some foods. Bulking agents such as guar, pectin, and fiber are used as energy diluents in processed foods. All of these pseudonutrients can effectively reduce the energy intake when incorporated into a well-balanced diet that is energy restricted. This will help the overweight individual lose excess fat.

Bariatric Surgery

Several surgical procedures have been developed to help the obese person lose weight. The first is called *liposuction* and involves the removal of a localized fat mass from a discrete part of the body. It cannot remove large amounts of fat but can be used to reduce/remove small fat deposits from areas that the individual finds objectionable. Liposuction can be used to remove a small fat pad that forms under the chin, for example. It was thought that it might be useful to remove belly fat, but subsequent experience with this use was found to be fraught with danger. The procedure uses a small incision through which a tube is inserted. Fluid is pumped in and the fat is sucked out. When used in the abdominal area, the surgeon cannot see what is being sucked; it is possible that instead of the sucking tube being placed in the middle of a discrete fat pad, it might be inadvertently placed near a portion of the intestine. If the intestine was lying close to the abdominal wall, this would be disastrous. Without knowing where the suction tip is actually placed, the intestine could be injured. Intestinal contents could leak out into the peritoneal cavity, and due to the fact that intestinal contents are rich with flora, peritonitis could develop. Nonetheless, liposuction has its uses when discrete fat pads can be removed. Fat pads such as those under the chin can successfully be removed with few side effects. A second surgical procedure to treat obesity is the lap band procedure. In this procedure an apparatus is placed around the upper part of the stomach. The apparatus has an adjustable band that can be tightened or loosened as needed. The apparatus reduces the storage capacity of the stomach, giving the individual less area for food. This elicits a feeling of satiety and reduces the amount of food consumed. The net result is a reduction in energy intake (that hopefully results in a negative energy balance), which, as described previously, reduces the body fat stores. If the lap band apparatus is used in conjunction with an exercise program, the weight loss will involve an increase in muscle mass and a decrease in fat store.

Last is a more radical surgical procedure, *gastric bypass*. In this procedure a large portion of the stomach is bypassed. It is left in place but simply does not receive any food. A small portion of the stomach (the upper portion that is connected to the esophagus) is then joined to the middle part of the small intestine. Because the stomach is severely reduced in size, the individual can consume only *very* small portions of food at any one time. This creates a semistarvation situation and large amounts of the fat store are lost. There are a number of metabolic problems associated with this large trauma. First of all, there is the immediate catabolic hormone response to the trauma of the surgery. These hormones are those that stimulate the breakdown of fat and to some extent the breakdown of protein. Glycogen stores, of which there are very little compared to the fat stores, are raided as well. The metabolic response to the surgical trauma accounts for much of the initial weight loss, and the individual must be able to withstand this metabolic response. Careful scrutiny of the prospective patient is absolutely essential to the success of the surgery.

After the patient has recovered from the trauma of the surgery, the fat loss continues, but at a somewhat reduced rate. The patient is still in negative energy balance and is definitely oxidizing the excess fat store. However, as time passes, the small residual stomach expands to allow the patient to increase the amount of food that can be consumed at any one time. Eventually, a new homeostasis is established with a new body weight (with an associated reduced fat store) that is then maintained. In some patients the residual stomach expands far more than expected and some of these patients begin to develop a new fat store. In other patients there are problems of anemia because the residual stomach that was connected to the middle portion of the intestine did not include the cells that produce and release the intrinsic factor needed for the absorption of vitamin B_{12}. Anemia in these patients develops and must be treated with B_{12} injections. Mineral absorption could also be reduced because of inadequate acidification of the food or because there is insufficient area for absorption. Most of the digestive enzymes are produced within the portion of the intestine that is bypassed, so this could affect nutrient absorption. All of these problems subsequent to the surgery can be managed if the patient is given good follow-up care.

Conclusion

While the treatment of obesity is the subject of continuing research, the optimal plan is to develop a strategy whereby treatment of excess body fat stores is unnecessary; that is, excess fat gain is avoided through monitoring food intake and maintenance of an active lifestyle. The goal is to actively maintain normal weight homeostasis. The case studies in this chapter are designed to help you understand how homeostasis can be perturbed, and the consequences of such perturbations.

Learning Activity 3.1: Keeping a Food Diary

The homeostatic regulation of body weight includes the regulation of food intake as well as the activity of the individual. How do you know what you eat? The simplest way is to keep a food diary for 3 days. Write down everything you eat and drink. Record the quantities of these foods. Start with breakfast and include all snacks and beverages. At first you will have to use a measuring cup and maybe a food scale. A food scale can be purchased very cheaply at a drug store or grocery store pharmacy. They usually cost $3–4. After a while your eye will be trained and you will be able to estimate very closely the quantity of what you are eating. After you have made a 3-day record, write down all the energy values of these foods. You can use the Web to acquire this information from tables of food composition. There are also computer programs available, and if your college has these, use them. You should then add up all the energy values of the foods you have consumed over the 3-day period and divide by three. That will give you a pretty good estimate of what you usually consume. Don't forget to include a weekend day in your 3-day record. Sometimes weekends differ. Perhaps you like to sleep late and go to brunch around 11 a.m. This might mean you skip both breakfast and lunch and then go out with friends for supper. This would be different from your Monday through Friday routine.

After you have done this you will see how much you are eating, and if you are gaining or losing weight you might want to adjust your food intake accordingly.

Record	*Meal*	*Food Item*	*Quantity*	*Energy Content (Kilocalories)*
Day 1				
	Breakfast			
	Lunch			
	Dinner			
	Snacks			
Day 2				
	Breakfast			
	Lunch			
	Dinner			
	Snacks			
Day 3				
	Breakfast			
	Lunch			
	Dinner			
	Snacks			

Case Study 3.1: Marcus Wants to Stop Gaining Weight

Marcus is a member of his high school wrestling team. He was 5′6″ tall, weighed 135 pounds, and was 14 years old at the beginning of his sophomore year. At this time he began gaining small amounts of weight. Although at first this did not seem a very serious situation, over time Marcus became concerned that he might have to move up to the next weight class, where he thought he might be less competitive. Marcus began trying a variety of methods to keep his weight down while still preserving his hard-won muscle tissue. His methods included weight work in the gym, aerobic work such as running and swimming, taking saunas, fasting for a day before competition weigh-in, and eating a high-protein diet recommend by the local diet center. Although these methods reduced his weight gain, Marcus was not satisfied. He wanted to stay in his 135–145 weight class for wrestling. He decided to try the diet pills that his mother and sister used. This seemed to work for a few weeks, but Marcus found that the diet pills were not suppressing his appetite. He was still very hungry. He stopped taking them but he decided to make himself vomit the food he ate so that this food would not have an effect on his weight. He found that he could eat enough to feel satisfied, and if he then vomited all this food, he could suppress weight gain. Although he finished the season in the weight class he desired, by spring he had gained several inches in height and he worried that through the summer he might not remain in the weight class he wanted to be in. He thought about the summer and realized that it would be a long hard slog against weight gain, so Marcus continued to induce himself to vomit. He also continued his strenuous exercise program with the goal of increasing muscle strength. He stopped consuming the high-protein drink recommended by the food store. However, during the summer a routine dental appointment revealed erosion of Marcus's tooth enamel and enlargement of his salivary glands. At the same time, Marcus complained to his dentist of constant muscle cramps at unexpected times that were hard to resolve. The dentist recognized the signs of bulimia nervosa (self-induced vomiting) and discussed this with Marcus and his father. Marcus admitted that he had been inducing vomiting to control his weight. The dentist recommended that Marcus see the family physician for a physical. The physician observed slight dehydration and esophageal inflammation and noted that Marcus's weight was only 70% of the expected weight for his height. Bulimia nervosa was confirmed but Marcus refused to see the psychologist as recommended and said that he would stop his self-induced vomiting instead.

Marcus did stop his self-induced vomiting but then over the summer he gained some weight. When the gain was around 10 pounds he was seriously worried about entering his junior year as a wrestler in the next weight class. He convinced himself that he did not want to do this, so he decided to try laxatives as a form of weight control. He thought that this might avoid the health consequences of induced vomiting.

A few weeks into the new season, Marcus fractured his upper arm. The radiologist at the hospital noted that Marcus's bone density was low for his age and recommended a consult with his family physician. This time, a panel of tests demonstrated an electrolyte imbalance. His tissue potassium was low and the blood values likewise for chloride, potassium, sodium, magnesium, and calcium were abnormal. The blood workup showed that he was anemic, hypovolemic, and hypoprotenemic. More sophisticated bone density tests demonstrated that Marcus has osteomalacia. In addition, Marcus's EKG showed a cardiac arrhythmia. He was admitted to the local hospital for treatment and began counseling with a psychologist and a nutritionist with the goal of helping Marcus understand that his condition was induced by his forced vomiting and then his use of laxatives coupled with excess exercise.

Problem Analysis and Resolution

Based on this case study, your textbook, and other outside sources, answer the following questions:

1. Why was Marcus diagnosed with bulimia nervosa rather than anorexia nervosa? (What is the difference between these two conditions?)

2. Why was Marcus having so much trouble with muscle cramps at unexpected times?

3. Explain why Marcus was dehydrated. Why was he also hypokalemic?

4. Suppose Marcus had never tried anything but the diet pills and laxatives. Would his symptoms be any different? What would still be the same?

5. Why was Marcus gaining weight despite his efforts to avoid weight gain? Speculate on the composition of the weight gain. (Was it fat? Fat and protein? Water? Mineral? All of these? Why?)

6. What strategies would you suggest to help Marcus recover?

Case Study 3.2: Susie's Goldfish Jumps Out of the Bowl

Susie had a goldfish as a pet. One day the goldfish jumped out of its bowl and was not discovered for several hours. Susie was devastated, but her mom, being a rather practical soul, suggested that the goldfish be returned to the bowl to see what would happen. Susie thought for sure that the fish was dead; after all, a fish needs to swim in water to get oxygen to its lungs and this fish had been oxygen deprived for several hours. Lo and behold, as soon as the fish was returned to the bowl it began to swim around as if nothing had happened. Susie was delighted!

Problem Analysis and Resolution

Based on your textbook and on other resources, answer the following questions:

1. Explain how the goldfish survived under these adverse conditions. What homeostatic mechanisms were at work here?

2. What is unique about a fish that allows it to survive when mammals deprived of oxygen cannot?

3. What metabolic end products does the fish produce in large quantities in this situation that mammals do not? (Mammals may produce small amounts of these end products in the course of their metabolism, but under oxygen deprivation they do not produce what the fish produces.)

Case Study 3.3: Beth Decides

Beth has struggled with her weight ever since she was a child. During grade school and high school, she gradually became used to being the "fat girl" in any group of friends. She adjusted well socially and did not pay attention to potential long-term complications of a life lived in an overburdened body. However, after the birth of her two children, she gained significantly more weight and no amount of dieting or exercise seemed to help. She became morbidly obese, more than 100 pounds over her ideal weight. At this point, Beth's family health history caught up with her.

About two years after the birth of her first child, Beth was diagnosed with type 2 diabetes (diabetes mellitus) and hypertension. Additionally, her blood work showed an elevated cholesterol level. She had trouble sleeping due to sleep apnea and had problems with acid reflux. Weight (excess body fat stores) became a serious problem. After researching the options for reducing her body weight, Beth makes an appointment with a bariatric surgeon. After a series of screening tests to ensure that she is an appropriate candidate for surgery, Beth has a gastric bypass.

Because gastric bypass is such a radical procedure, Beth is required by her physician to work closely with a dietician to plan and maintain a diet that provides appropriate nutrients and energy so that she can maintain her lifestyle.

Problem Analysis and Resolution

Based on the above story, answer the following questions:

1. Why has Beth developed type 2 diabetes?

2. Why was pregnancy a precipitating event for Beth's weight?

3. What options are there for Beth in her current condition? What are the benefits and risks of these options?

4. Why are osteoporosis and anemia often seen as side-effects of bypass surgery? Discuss the physiology of the system and how it is affected by the surgery in terms of explaining the secondary conditions that subsequently develop.

5. Suggest a diet and a lifestyle that would support Beth as she undergoes the surgery and recovers from same.

Case Study 3.4: Baby Bo Can't Get Enough

Bo's proud new Mom didn't realize that babies required quite so much food or diaper changing! At their regular 6-month checkup, she comments to Bo's pediatrician that Bo seems to nurse much more frequently than did her nieces. She has also noticed that his diaper needs changing much more frequently than she thinks it should (about every 30 minutes). She reports that because Bo needs to eat about every hour, she is having to supplement his diet with infant formula to meet Bo's demands. Since this sounded a bit excessive to the physician, a complete physical is performed. Results follow:

Vital Signs
Rectal temperature = 98.9° F (37.2°C)
Heart rate = 85 beats/min
Respiratory rate = 13 breaths/min
Weight loss since last visit

Reflexes
All within normal range, but slightly excitable

Skin and Mucous Membranes
Lack of skin turgor; sunken fontanel; mucous membranes dry

Blood
Hematocrit (Hct) = 59%
Serum sodium = 139 mEq/L
Serum potassium = 5 mEq/L
Serum bicarbonate = 21 mEq/L
Serum chloride = 109 mEq/L
ADH = elevated
BUN = 5 mg/dL

Urine
Specific gravity = 1.002; pH = 6.8
Glucose, proteins, lipids, blood cells all absent

Additional testing included a water deprivation test, which resulted in no change in urine osmolarity.

Problem Analysis and Resolution

1. Suggest Bo's problem. Describe how you arrived at your suggestion using the information above.

2. Bo's problem usually is the result of a genetic error. Describe this error and the result-ing change to his physiological management of fluids and electrolytes.

3. Is dietary management of Bo's condition possible? If so, how is this done? Will he need additional pharmaceutical intervention?

4. Suppose Bo's blood work had demonstrated no measurable amounts of antidiuretic hormone (ADH). Does this result suggest a different source for Bo's problem?

Case Study 3.5: Discovering a Concentration Camp

After Germany surrendered at the end of World War II, the allied troops spread out over the territory and much to their dismay discovered numerous camps for prisoners of war and for people the Germans thought should not be citizens of their country. When the troops entered these camps, they found numerous starving people. They immediately emptied their backpacks of any food they possessed and gave it to the ex-prisoners. However, medical personnel caught up with the troops and demanded the return of the food, saying that the troops were going to kill these survivors if all that food was consumed.

Problem Analysis and Resolution

1. Why did the medical people demand that the troops not give food to these hungry people? Explain the homeostatic mechanisms operating that ensured survival in these people. Why would a lot of food kill them?

2. What do you suppose would be the most appropriate treatment for these survivors? Justify these treatments.

chapter 4

Blood

Blood is the medium for the transport of the needed essentials of life. The blood circulates within a closed system called the vascular system. Contained by the blood are the red blood cells (the erythrocytes), the white cells (including antibodies and macrophages), platelets, fibrin, clotting factors, various metabolites, electrolytes, various hormones and cytokines, various lipids, and eicosanoids. Some of these are listed in Table 4.1. Chapter 1 contains several tables giving the normal levels of some of these components. As can be seen, the blood is a rich supplier of everything the body needs to stay alive and to respond to the external environment. The blood serves a fundamental role in the maintenance of homeostasis and, because it is a readily accessible tissue, it has been much studied. The process of blood clotting has been revealed through the study of clotting components; the identification of small proteins that serve as messengers (the cytokines) has been possible because blood samples can be drawn and studied in response to a variety of treatments. The same is also true for studies of the function of the eicosanoids, hormones, and metabolic flux. We have learned so much about the function of the body through studies of the various components of blood.

Of interest to the nutritionist is the red blood cell, the erythrocyte. Its function is quite simple. It is responsible for delivering oxygen to all the cells of the body and exchanging that oxygen for carbon dioxide. The carbon dioxide is then delivered to the lungs for release via the expired air. The erythrocyte is a short-lived cell with a half-life of about 60 days. Replacement cells must be made constantly through the process of hematopoiesis. Hematopoiesis is responsible for all of the blood cells (white cells, platelets, and red cells) and takes place in the pluripotent stem cells of the bone marrow. Erythropoiesis is solely responsible for the red cell synthesis through a process of proliferation and differentiation. It is dependent on an intact bone marrow environment and on a cascade or network of cytokines, growth factors, and nutrients. The main function of the red cell is to carry oxygen to all cells of the body and exchange it for carbon dioxide. A shortfall in the number of red cells or in its oxygen-carrying capacity is called *anemia*. Table 4.2 lists the nutrients important to normal red cell production. It is of interest to note that many of the symptoms of malnutrition include anemia. This is because red blood cells are among the shortest lived cells in the body and abnormalities in them will develop and be noticeable long before changes in other cell types are observed.

Causes of Nutritional Anemia

Among the most common reasons for anemia is iron deficiency. This is especially true for adult menstruating females whose diets can be iron poor. Iron is poorly absorbed, and many diets, especially those consumed by third-world populations, are iron poor. Diets that contain mainly whole grain cereals and legumes contain only nonheme iron, which is poorly absorbed. Assessment of deficiency includes the determination of levels of tissue ferritin, transferrin, receptor activity, heme iron, red cell number, and hemoglobin levels.

Table 4.1 Some Blood Components

Albumin
Globulins and other glycoproteins
Lipoproteins
Fibrinogen and coagulation factors
Platelets
Hemoglobin (in erythrocytes)
Transferrin
Ceruloplasmin
Steroid binding proteins
Retinol binding proteins
Thyroid binding proteins
Erythrocytes
Hormones
Cytokines
Eicosanoids
B lymphocytes containing immunoglobulins
T lymphocytes containing cell-mediated immunologic processes
Complement system components (~20 different proteins)
Electrolytes

The availability of iron from food depends on its source. Soybean protein, for example, contains an inhibitor of iron uptake. Diets such as those in Asia contain numerous soybean products, and iron absorption is adversely affected by this soybean inhibitor. Tannins, phytates, certain fibers (not cellulose), carbonates, phosphates, and low protein diets also adversely affect the apparent absorption of iron. In contrast, ascorbic acid, fructose, citric acid, high animal protein foods, lysine, histidine, cysteine, methionine, and natural chelates, that is, heme, all enhance the apparent absorption of iron. Zinc and manganese reduce iron uptake by about 30–50% and 10–40%, respectively. Excess iron reduces zinc uptake by 13–22%. Stearic acid, one of the main fatty acids in meat, also enhances iron uptake. Two types of iron are present in food: heme iron, which is found principally in animal products, and nonheme iron, which is inorganic iron bound to various proteins in the plant. Most of the iron in the diet, usually greater than 85%, is present in the nonheme form. The absorption of nonheme iron is strongly influenced by its solubility in the upper part of the intestine. Absorption of nonheme iron depends on the composition of the meal and is subject to enhancers of absorption such as animal protein and by reducing agents such as vitamin C. Heme iron, however, is absorbed more efficiently. It is not subject to

Table 4.2 Nutrients Needed for Red Cell Production

Protein
Energy
Vitamins E, A, B_6, B_{12}
Folacin
Iron, copper, zinc
Riboflavin
Niacin

these enhancers. Although heme iron accounts for a smaller proportion of iron in the diet, it provides quantitatively more iron to the body than dietary nonheme iron.

The regulation of iron entry into the body takes place in the mucosal cells of the small intestine. Its iron gate is very sensitive to the iron stores, so if the iron stores are low, which is true for most women and children, the intestinal mucosa takes up iron and increases the proportion absorbed from the diet. However, if the body is replete with iron, as is typical of healthy men and postmenopausal women, then the percentage of iron absorbed is low. This mechanism offers some protection against iron overload. In infancy, lactoferrin, an iron-binding protein in human milk, promotes the absorption of iron through lactoferrin receptors on the surface of the intestinal mucosa of infants. This may explain why iron is well absorbed from human milk. Milk is not usually considered a good source of iron, but for the breast-fed infant this lactoferrin–iron mechanism prevents deficiency from developing. As the infant matures, however, this mechanism becomes inadequate.

Iron uptake by the gut, iron use and reuse, and iron loss constitutes a system that for all intents and purposes is a closed system. The gain through the gut is very inefficient and there is virtually no mechanism aside from blood loss that rids the body of its iron excess. The total iron content of the body averages 4.0 g in men and 2.6 g in women. Hemoglobin is the most abundant and easily sampled of the heme proteins and accounts for greater than 65% of body iron. Transferrin is the iron-transport protein that carries the iron ion between the sites of its absorption, storage, and utilization. It binds two atoms of ferric iron per mole. Transferrin is synthesized in the liver, brain, and testes, as well as other tissues. The amount of transferrin synthesized is inversely related to the iron supply. In times of low intake, more transferrin is produced so as to optimize iron availability.

Once iron enters the cell, it is chelated to a protein that is then called ferritin. This reaction represents the ultimate destination for the majority of the iron that enters the cell. Hemosiderin is a form of denatured ferritin and contains about one-third of the iron store in the body. Ferritin also serves as a zinc detoxicant and a zinc ion donor. This is important in instances where a zinc overload has occurred. The hormone hepciden is a key regulator of iron balance. When elevated it serves to increase iron in macrophages and decrease gastrointestinal iron uptake. The synthesis of hepcidin is induced by infection, inflammation, and elevated iron intake. Low levels of hepcidin are associated with anemia, hypoxia, iron deficiency, and hereditary hemochromatosis. In response to inflammation, IL6 levels rise followed by rises in hepcidin. Hepcidin inhibits iron release by the macrophages and this inhibition results in a fall in serum iron. The export of iron from enterocytes and macrophages is mediated by ferroportin. Hepcidin acts by binding ferroportin on the plasma membranes causing it to be internalized and degraded. This increases enterocyte iron, which eventually passes this into the lumen of the gastrointestinal tract. Hepcidin deficiency seems to be the basis for hemochromatosis, a condition of excess iron in the blood.

Since the lifetime of a red cell is about 120 days in humans (half-life of ~60 days), the flow of iron through the plasma space amounts to about 25–30 mg/day in the adult (about 0.5 mg/kg body weight). This amount of iron corresponds to the degradation of about 1% of the circulating hemoglobin mass per day. Iron is conserved in the body in males and postmenopausal females to a great degree, only 10% being lost per year in normal men, or about 1 mg/day. This loss of 1 mg/day has to be made up by absorption of iron from the diet, which is only about 10% efficient, requiring about 10 mg of dietary iron/day. In menstruating females the loss is increased to 2 mg/day, which means that the intake and absorption of iron must be increased or these females will develop iron deficiency.

Upon destruction, the normal red cell is taken up by the reticulo-endothelial system and the hemoglobin is degraded into bile pigments and ferric iron. The ferric ion enters the transferrin pool and is recirculated. Thus, the turnover of iron within the body is 10–20 times the amount absorbed. A similar small amount, ~1 mg/d, is lost by the sloughing of gastrointestinal cells and by skin cells. Fecal losses of iron are about 0.6 mg/day. Urinary losses are essentially nil.

In menstruating women, or in individuals with hemorrhage, the iron losses can be considerable and anemia can occur as a result of menstrual losses or bleeding. This is the basis for the chlorosis (chronic hypochromic microcytic anemia) observed in adolescent girls. This symptom is one of the first characteristics associated with a nutrient deficiency and was first identified as iron deficiency in the 17th century. Females, during the child-bearing years, must replace the iron lost in menstrual blood, which over a month amounts to about 1.4 mg/day. During infancy and childhood, about 40 mg of iron are required for the production of essential iron compounds associated with the gain of 1 kg of new tissue. Obviously the iron needs are great in the rapid growth phases of infancy and adolescence. The needs of pregnant women are also great because during pregnancy a total of about 1.0 g of iron is needed to cover the growth need of the fetus and that of the mother as she prepares for delivery and lactation. It is difficult to obtain this amount of iron from the usual diet. It is estimated that about 27 mg/day of elemental iron is needed in the diet to provide sufficient iron to the pregnant female.

The appearance of clinical iron deficiency anemia occurs in three stages. The first involves depletion of iron stores as measured by decrease in serum ferritin, which reflects the ferritin supply (iron stores) in the body, without loss of essential iron compounds and without any evidence of anemia. The second stage is characterized by biochemical changes that reflect the lack of iron sufficient for the normal production of hemoglobin and other iron compounds. This is indicated by a decrease in transferrin saturation levels and an increase in erythrocyte protophyrin—so-called iron deficiency without anemia. In the final stage, the appearance of iron deficiency anemia occurs with depressed hemoglobin production and a change in the mean corpuscular volume of the red blood cells to produce a microcytic hypochromic anemia (see Table 4.3). This is expressed clinically as pallor and weakness. There are also changes in the nails, which take on a spoon shape when the iron deficient state is severe.

Pharmacological Treatment of Iron Deficiency

The treatment of iron deficiency anemia is a pharmacological activity and involves giving large doses of iron, usually equivalent to 60 mg of elemental iron or 300 mg of ferrous sulfate, once or twice a day. It is usually given between meals to minimize gastrointestinal side effects. Fortunately, the smaller the dose and the more severe the anemia, the greater will be the percentage of iron absorbed. This treatment is usually continued for 2 to 3 months to normalize hemoglobin levels and iron stores. These should be monitored until satisfactory values are obtained.

Toxicology of Iron Overload

Iron toxicity is a result of excess iron intake. This can occur acutely in children who ingest iron pills or iron-vitamin supplements not realizing that they can be toxic. Severe iron poisoning is characterized by damage to the intestine with bloody diarrhea, vomiting, acidosis, and sometimes liver failure. Effective treatment includes induced emesis

Table 4.3 Normal Blood Values for Measurements Made to Assess the Presence of Anemia

Measurement	Normal Values	Iron Deficiency	Chronic Disease	B_{12} or Folic Acid Deficiency
Red blood cells	Males: 4.6–6.2 (million/cu mm); Females: 4.2–5.4	Low	Low	Low
Hemoglobin (g/dL)	Males: 14–18; Females: 12–16	Low	Low	Low
Hematocrit (vol %)	Males: 40–54%; Females: 37–47%	Low	Low	Low
Serum iron	60–280 ug/dL	Low	Low	Normal
TIBC[a]	250–425 ug/dL	High	Low	Normal
Ferritin	Less than 12	Normal	Normal	
Percent sat.	90–100%	Low	Normal to high	Normal
Hypochromia	No	Yes	Slight	None
Microcytes	Few	Many	Slight	Few
Macrocytes	Few	Few	None	Many
RDW (RBC size)	High	High	Normal to low	Very high
Red cell folate	>360 nmol/L	Normal	315–358	<315
Serum folate	>13.5 mg/mL	Normal	Normal	Low (<6.7)
Serum B_{12}	200–900 pg/mL	Normal	Normal	Low
MCV[b]	82–92 cu m	<80	Normal	>80–100

[a] Indirect measure of serum transferrin; iron binding capacity.
[b] Mean cell volume. When volume increases, the size of the red cell increases ($\uparrow$ % of megaloblasts).

(vomiting), food and electrolyte treatment to prevent shock, and the use of iron chelating agents to bind the iron. This treatment has substantially decreased the mortality from about 50% in 1950 to less than a few percent in recent years.

Other Nutrients and Anemia

As mentioned in the discussion of iron homeostasis, other minerals are involved in the prevention of nutritional anemia. Copper serves to enhance iron absorption, and zinc is needed as an essential cofactor for numerous enzymes, some of which are involved in iron homeostasis and some are involved in erythropoiesis as well as for protein synthesis. Cobalt, as an essential ingredient of vitamin B_{12}, is also an important mineral to prevent anemia. Vegetarians are at risk for developing pernicious anemia because vitamin B_{12} is found in foods of animal origin. Humans do not synthesize this vitamin as do the flora found in the ruminant. While vegetarians obtain sufficient cobalt, they may be vitamin B_{12}-deficient. Cobalt has no known function aside from its central action in vitamin B_{12} function. Many vitamin deficiency states have anemia as a symptom. This is because they have roles in either enhancing iron absorption (see previously) or because they have roles as coenzymes in the synthesis of DNA, RNA, and proteins that are needed in erythropoiesis. Included in this group of micronutrients are thiamin, riboflavin, niacin, pyridoxine, folacin, vitamin B_{12}, and biotin. Folacin and vitamin B_{12} have roles in red cell production and maturation. If either is in short supply, characteristic changes in the number and size of the red cells in the blood will be observed (see Table 4.3).

Non-Nutritional Anemia

A number of non-nutritional reasons for anemia exist. These include excessive blood loss (hemorrhage), drug-induced red cell destruction, and several genetic diseases: thalassemia, sickle cell anemia, and hemolytic anemia. The first two disorders are due to mutations in the genes for the globin molecules in hemoglobin. Hemolytic anemia can be due to mutations in the gene for red cell glucose 6-phosphate dehydrogenase or due to a mutation in the gene for red cell pyruvate kinase. More than 300 variants of the gene for the dehydrogenase have been identified. Usually this mutation is silent. That is, the individual is unaware that there is a problem with this enzyme. It is only after the person is given one of the sulfa drugs or one of the quinine drugs that the problem develops. When this occurs, the red cell loses its ability to maintain its redox state, and the cell falls apart, or hemolyzes. Hence the term, hemolytic anemia.

   Some toxic conditions can also cause anemia. Lead poisoning typically is characterized by anemia. Exposure to pesticides and to solvents can cause anemia. Primarily, this anemia is due to an effect of these toxic substances on the system that maintains the redox state of the cell or on the oxygen carrying hemoglobin within the cell.

Blood Groups

On the surface of the red cell are antigens. Not all people have the same antigens on their red blood cell membranes. People have been grouped into those who have type A antigens, those who have type B antigens, those who have neither A or B antigens, and those who have both A and B antigens. These are the A, B, AB, and O blood groups. These groups are important to know for the safety of blood transfusions. Should an A be transfused with B blood, serious consequences could follow. Anaphalactic shock as well as some other problems such as hemolysis of the red cells will develop. Superimposed on these blood groups are cells with a D antigen (called the Rh factor). If this antigen is present on the red cell membrane, the people with this red cell characteristic are classed as Rh+. Those without this factor are classed as Rh–. Usually Rh status is determined at the same time as the ABO grouping, and everyone should know his/her blood type. The Rh factor, however, has some serious consideration as an obstetric problem. If the mother is Rh– and the father is positive, the embryo/fetus could be positive. Since there is some transfer of blood components across the placenta, antibodies to the Rh factor could be raised in the mother. These would be transferred to the unborn child. When this incompatibility develops, the red blood cells of the unborn child could lyse (fall apart) and the child could die in utero. Many times, however, the child is born and this incompatibility is discovered. At this point the only option is to completely replace the infant's blood supply with Rh– blood. In many instances, the first-born child of an Rh– mother is normal and the incompatibility problem is not encountered. However, with subsequent pregnancies there can be problems. The mother has been sensitized by her first child and therefore has an antigen–antibody reaction already in place. If the second child is also Rh+ the situation is much worse than when the first child was in the womb. If the second child is Rh–, then few problems will be encountered. If both parents are Rh–, then none of the above applies. However, this is unlikely since only 15% of the population is Rh–.

Blood Clotting

The clotting of blood seals an opening in the skin and thus prevents pathogens from entering the body. It is a special defense mechanism that is used when injury occurs. It occurs via a cascade mechanism as shown in Figure 4.1. As can be seen, vitamin K is essential for normal blood clotting. It is needed in three places. These are places in the cascade where the calcium ion is involved. Vitamin K serves to stimulate the post-translational carboxylation of these proteins. In doing so it substantially increases the calcium binding capability of these proteins, and this calcium binding is essential to clot formation.

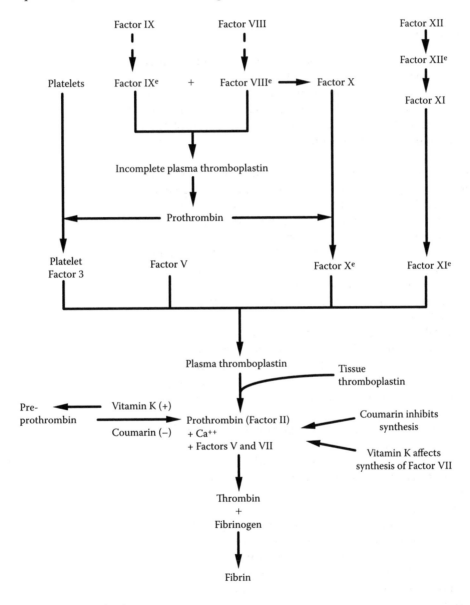

Figure 4.1 Formation of a clot.

There are instances when the formation of a clot is not desirable, as occurs in cardiovascular disease. People with cardiovascular disease have increased clot formation, and these clots can interfere with blood flow. To inhibit clot formation, people with cardiovascular disease are often prescribed anticlotting drugs. Aspirin in low doses is often coupled with dicumerol, an anti-vitamin K. Aspirin inhibits platelet activity. Other anticlotting drugs have also been developed. All of these drugs must be closely monitored, as the range of their effectiveness is narrow. Too much of these agents can cause excess bleeding. People taking these medications will notice an increase in the number of bruises that occur with little provocation.

White Cells

The cellular components of blood that are not red blood cells include the platelets and a whole collection of cells that fight infection. These are the white cells, which contain a variety of immunoglobulins. Leukocytes, neutrophils, and lymphocytes (both T and B lymphocytes) are white cells. Neutrophils are important to the body's defense against bacterial infection. Neutrophils, along with other macrophages, phagocytose bacteria. They surround the bacteria and engulf them and then, using an active peroxide producing system, destroy the bacteria.

Often, the physician will order a white cell differential count to determine whether an infection is present. The differential count will give an estimate of how many neutrophils, eosinophils, leukocytes, and so forth are present in the blood. Antibacterial or antiviral drugs can then be prescribed depending on the nature of the infection. It should be noted that there are very few really effective antiviral drugs. Most antibiotics are, in fact, antibacterial drugs rather than drugs that combat all pathogens. Each of the drugs available to the physician acts on certain pathogens but not on all pathogens; likewise, certain pathogens will respond to some drugs but not to others. Thus, when you have the common cold, a condition usually caused by a virus, antibacterial drugs will be of little use.

A number of diseases involving the white cell population exist. Much attention has been given to acquired immune deficiency syndrome (AIDS). This disease is thought to have arisen in Africa through the consumption of monkey brains. It was considered a zoonotic disease when it first appeared in the human population, but now the disease is passed from human to human when body fluids are exchanged. It involves the loss of the body's ability to produce antibodies to pathogens. Individuals with full-blown AIDS cannot fight off these pathogens because of their compromised immune system. The cause of death of an AIDS patient is sometimes something that would be of a minor concern to an unaffected person. It could be a viral infection or Karposi's sarcoma or pneumonia. There has been some progress in developing drugs to combat AIDS and techniques to manage the problems associated with AIDS, but none of these has cured the condition.

Other conditions involving the white cell population include the leukemias and the lymphomas. These are diagnosed when very high levels of these types of white cells are detected in the blood. There are several varieties of each of these diseases; however, common to all of them is an explosion in the number of these particular white cells in the blood. Both the leukemias and the lymphomas are considered as members of the cancer disease family.

Blood Pressure

Blood pressure is defined as the pressure exerted on the vascular tree by the blood within it in response to the contractions and relaxations of the heart muscle. When the heart contracts (systole), blood is forced out of the ventricles into the major arteries, arterioles, and thence into the peripheral blood supply. The vascular tree expands to allow this pulse of blood to flow through it. Then, when the heart relaxes (diastole) before the next contraction, the vascular tree contracts so that the blood can return to the heart for the next push forward through the next contraction. This periodic ebb and flow of the blood through the vascular system can be monitored through the measurement of blood pressure as mm mercury. Blood pressure is expressed as a fraction with the systolic pressure on top and the diastolic pressure on the bottom. A reading of 120/80 is considered normal. Hypertension, sometimes called *high blood pressure*, occurs when the vascular system does not relax sufficiently between heart beats. This may be due to a loss of elasticity of the vascular tree or may be due to other factors that appear to inhibit such relaxation. Low blood pressure, or hypotension, is the reverse. In this situation the vascular tree is over-relaxed and the blood flow is reduced. Hypotension can develop in times of hemorrhage, in response to malnutrition, as a result of overmedication, and due to an electrolyte imbalance.

As mentioned above, both nutritional and genetic factors regulate blood pressure. There is an interplay between the hormones that regulate blood pressure and electrolyte balance. Shown in Figure 4.2 is a diagram illustrating the hormones involved in the regulation of blood pressure. If any of these factors is out of balance, changes in blood pressure will follow.

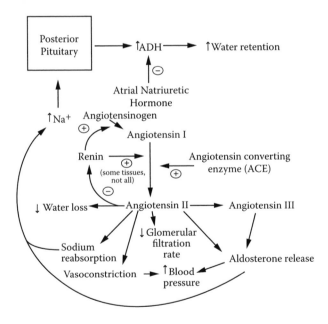

Figure 4.2 Blood pressure is under hormonal control. Abbreviation used: ADH, antidiuretic hormone.

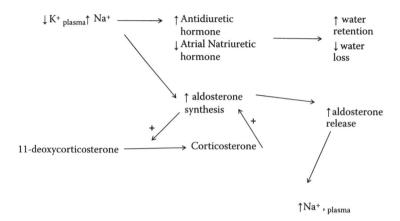

Figure 4.3 Changing potassium and sodium levels in the blood affects water balance and blood pressure.

As shown in Figure 4.2, there are points where blood pressure can be altered pharmacologically. For example, people with hypertension can be prescribed an angiotensin conversion inhibitor (ACE inhibitor). This lowers blood pressure by inhibiting the conversion of angiotensin I to angiotensin II. Other drugs target other points in the hormonal regulation of blood pressure. Hypertension has been linked to an increased risk for heart disease and stroke. Often, people with hypertension are asked to reduce their sodium intake.

The ratio of potassium to sodium has effects on water balance and on blood pressure. Figure 4.3 illustrates this in a very simplistic manner. Reducing sodium intake alters the ratio of sodium to potassium and in turn helps to lower blood pressure. There is also an association of hypertension with the consumption of dairy foods. Those individuals who regularly include milk, cheese, and other dairy products tend to have less hypertension than do those who abstain from these products. Dairy products are rich sources of calcium and magnesium, but whether these minerals are responsible for hypertension reduction is not known. Diuretics likewise can lower blood pressure and these are sometimes prescribed. Unfortunately, diuretics increase the loss of potassium and some researchers have proposed that high potassium intakes are beneficial with respect to the reduction of risk for hypertension. Last, excess body weight has a negative impact on blood pressure. Obese people are much more likely to develop hypertension than are thin people or people of normal body weight. Physical activity can help reduce the excess fat store and physically active people are less likely to develop hypertension than sedentary people.

Learning Activity 4.1: Your Nutritional Status

Using the food diary you constructed for Learning Activity 3.1, calculate estimates of your daily mineral and vitamin intake. Compare this value to those recommended for your age and gender. Go to the Web site, www.nap.edu, to obtain your daily recommended intakes for the micronutrients and then create a two-bar graph for each of the essential vitamins and minerals. One bar should be your intake and the second one (next to it) should be that recommended for you. For any of the micronutrients where there is more than a 10% difference, show how you are going to alter your food intake to erase this difference. The difference can be on either the plus side or the negative side. Do not include your intake of micronutrients via a vitamin/mineral supplement. If you take a supplement, you should look at the above bar graphs to determine whether you need to take this supplement or perhaps select another type of supplement. Show this comparison and list your conclusions.

Case Study 4.1: Cynthia Has an Automobile Accident

Cynthia is a 20-year-old college student. One night after a party at her boyfriend's fraternity house, she decided to drive to her parents' home for the weekend. It was late Friday and there was beer as well as some snack food at the party. Cynthia was not driving under the influence, but being tired she was not as alert as she should have been. The driving conditions were not ideal: There had been a light misty rain and it was foggy in places. As Cynthia was traveling around a curve, an oncoming car with headlights on high beam suddenly appeared. Cynthia tried to escape a collision but she was unsuccessful, and the two cars met head on. Fortunately, both cars were being driven cautiously and relatively slowly so neither driver was killed. Both were seriously injured. Both were transported to the local hospital by ambulance. Both suffered fractures and they both lost blood. Cynthia was worse off than the other driver. The other driver was a 35-year-old male.

Problem Analysis and Resolution

1. Suppose you were the physician in the emergency room that received these two drivers. What would you do first and then what would you consider for the recuperative phase?

2. Justify your actions and recuperative plan.

Case Study 4.2: Nebraska Pioneer Women

In the late 1800s many young couples homesteaded in the plains states of Kansas, Iowa, Nebraska, the Dakotas, and so forth. Some had migrated from the east with very few resources and very little farming experience. The land was free if you could "prove it up"—that is, if you lived and farmed the land you homesteaded for a set period of time. Some of these couples built dug-out homes or sod homes, and cooked on an open fire with very little cooking equipment. They ate what they grew and sometimes did not have very much to eat between harvests and the gathering of wild plants and the killing of wild animals. Those who had greater resources would have cast-iron cooking pots and were able from time to time to buy needed staples.

After living out on the prairie for months at a time, the women would become unable to work and maintain their households. They became pale, listless, and weak. They would be taken into the nearby towns for rest and recuperation. After a month or two they usually "perked up" and were able to return to their homesteads.

Problem Analysis and Resolution

1. How would you explain what was happening to these women?

2. What strategies could have prevented some of these problems?

Case Study 4.3: Maureen Decides to Adopt Vegetarianism

Maureen has always been a soft-hearted individual. She loves all manner of creatures and when she went away to college, she became aware of the fact that beef, lamb, chicken, and even pork chops came from living creatures, and she hated the idea that these creatures were killed to provide food for her. So, she decided that she would no longer eat meat; she would eat only fruits and vegetables. She would, however, continue to enjoy small amounts of cheese, eggs, and milk.

This diet seemed to be very satisfying, but after about 6 months of vegetarianism she began to feel less energetic than she used to feel. She decided that she should have a check-up, and her doctor ordered a blood workup. He discovered that she was anemic. She had far fewer than normal red cells, and many of these cells were very small or were very large immature ones.

Problem Analysis and Resolution

1. What did the doctor conclude about Maureen?

2. What treatment do you think he administered?

3. What recommendations did he make?

chapter 5

You Are What You Eat

It should come as no surprise that an individual's health status is a reflection of the kinds and amounts of food that person consumes on a regular basis. There are numerous reasons why people choose the foods they eat. Some choices, of course, are based in the culture and economic status of the consumer. Some choices are dictated by food availability and some are dictated by the consumer's ability to prepare the food for consumption. Knowing that physical health is dependent on an adequate diet, the federal government has devised a series of recommendations which should ensure that people who follow these recommendations are adequately nourished. The National Academy of Sciences Food and Nutrition Board has devised a table of recommended nutrient intakes (DRIs) that is revised on a regular basis. It can be accessed on the Web at www.nap.edu. This is very valuable information, because people consume food, not specific nutrients. They therefore need food intake recommendations that will satisfy their needs for the essential nutrients. Here, too, the federal government has developed a set of recommendations called *dietary guidelines*. Table 5.1 shows some of the Web sites available to help people understand what they need to eat. Web sites giving food composition are also provided in this table.

Dietary Guidelines

The dietary guidelines are designed to maximize the nutrient intake so as to promote health. They are updated on a regular basis so that the results of current research can be incorporated as appropriate into these guidelines. All federal, state, and local government-sponsored food programs such as food stamps, the school lunch/school breakfast programs, and the Women, Infants, and Children program (WIC) use these guidelines to develop program services. The guidelines provide advice on the food choices that promote health and reduce the risk of disease. The guidelines have been used to construct a graph that shows in a single picture the foods that Americans should include in their daily diets. This picture is in the form of a pyramid (MyPyramid). Those foods that should be consumed in the largest amount are at the bottom of the pyramid, while those foods that should be minimally consumed are at the top. MyPyramid was designed "to motivate consumers to make healthier choices and to ensure that this food guidance system reflects the latest nutrition science." Over the years the problems of malnutrition have shifted, and so the guidelines have shifted as well. In earlier times, nutritionists were concerned with inadequate nutrient intakes. This is still a concern, but in many Western countries with an ample food supply, there is a growing concern about excess intakes of energy-rich foods coupled with a decrease in physical activity.

Diet Assessment

How do we know what people eat? A number of techniques can be used to determine what and how much food is being consumed. One is the 24-hour recall. The subject is asked to recall what he/she ate yesterday. It is an estimate of actual intake. It depends on

Table 5.1 Web Sites for Information on Food Intake

Use	Web Address
Food composition	www.nal.usda.gov/fnic/foodcomp/data/ foods,82nutrients
Foods from India	www.unu.edu/unupress/unupbooks/80633Eoi.htm
Foods from Europe	Cost99/EUROFOODS:Inventory of European food composition
	food.ethz.ch/cost99db-inventory.htm
Foods, developing nations	www.fao.org/DOCREP/WOO73e/woo73eO6htm
Other food data	www.arborcom.com/frame/foodc.htm
Foods from McDonald's restaurants	www.mcdonalds.com
Food intake recommendations: DRI	www.nap.edu www.nal.usda.gov/fnic/etext/000105.html
Dietary guidelines	www.health.gov/dietary guidelines
Food pyramid	www.mypyramid.gov/tips resources/menus.html

the individual actually remembering what he/she consumed and how much. Investigators using this method to assess nutrient intakes of large groups of people will request that the subjects provide a detailed description of the food, including brand names if known, ingredients of mixed dishes, food preparation methods, and portion sizes. Prompts for quantification of portion size such as two- or three-dimensional food models or detailed food pictures are typically employed. Nutrient intake can then be estimated for the designated day or portion of the day with this level of detail. These estimations can provide information about the group, but this method is not appropriate for an individual nutrient intake evaluation or to predict individual-level health outcomes such as serum cholesterol levels. Because of intra-individual variation in intake, multiple recalls are needed to accurately estimate an individual's usual food (and nutrient) intake. A number of computer-based programs are available that allow for the determination of nutrient intake using food intake data.

Another method for determining food intake is the food record method (the diary method). In this instance, the subject writes down everything that is eaten and tries to estimate the amount eaten. Training in estimating portion size increases the reliability of the record, as does the use of measuring equipment (standardized measuring cups for volume measurements and scales for weight measurements). These food records are written accounts of the intake of the food and beverages consumed during a specified time period, usually 3, 5, or 7 days. It is a measure of actual intake and, like the 24-hour recall, is appropriate for estimating group means. Again, there are a number of computer programs designed to facilitate the nutrient intake analysis of these records. Some food companies will provide nutrient analysis of their products to help the consumer to make good food choices. In addition, federal law mandates that the nutrient content be provided on the labels of canned and frozen food products. By reading the labels the consumer can see the nutrient content and portion sizes of the food products. Some of these are deceiving because what the consumer perceives as a portion size might not be the same as what the food manufacturer puts on the label. As an example, the manufacturer might declare that ten 1" crackers are a serving size, while the consumer might believe that 20 crackers are a serving size. The consumer has to look carefully at the label to determine what constitutes a serving size and make calculations accordingly with respect to the nutrient content of the food product.

A third method for determining food intake is the food frequency questionnaire. These questionnaires (FFQs) are relatively easy to use, less expensive than other assessment methods, and easily adapted for population studies. A measure of usual intake can be used to rank respondents by intake levels and is useful for predicting health outcomes at both the group and individual level. Respondents report their usual intake over a defined period of time in the past year, month, or week, although frequency of intake on the previous day has also been assessed. The FFQ can be self administered, interviewer administered, or group administered. Respondents are asked to report frequency of consumption and sometimes portion size for a defined list of foods. FFQs can be classified as quantitative, semiquantitative, or nonquantitative. Data from nonquantitative FFQs are generally used to assess frequency of consumption of food; however, these frequencies may also be associated with standard portions to estimate nutrient intakes.

Diet histories can be used to assess the past diet of an individual in the form of usual meal patterns, food intake, and food preparation practices. This method requires an extensive interview by a skilled, knowledgeable person. The interviewer can use a standardized questionnaire to guide the interview or can have the subject fill out a questionnaire prior to or following the interview. The diet history thus acquired provides a measure of the usual intake of the target population that is appropriate for ranking individuals and for predicting general (but not specific) health outcomes. In contrast to other methods of dietary assessment, a diet history is usually more qualitative than quantitative, allowing detailed information about food preparation, eating habits, and food consumption to be collected by a highly trained interviewer.

A variant of the diet history interview is the observation method. This method is useful for assessing subjects who cannot communicate via a written record. This method is labor intensive and requires that the observer record every food item (and quantity) the subject consumes over a set period of time. This observation provides a measure of actual intake that is appropriate for estimating group means. Multiple observations are usually necessary to provide reliable measures of usual intake.

All of these dietary assessment methods have inherent errors but are useful for assessing populations on the whole. They can reveal interesting food consumption trends and can be used to predict future outcomes with respect to health and wellbeing. In contrast, nutrition assessment that uses physiological measures (e.g., height, weight, skinfold thicknesses, body water measurements, doubly labeled water measurements, serum micronutrients, and measures of body functions relevant to nutrition) does not rely on information provided by respondents. The results of these types of measurements are thus more independent compared to a respondent-based measure. Comparisons of physiological endpoints, such as blood nutrient levels, to dietary assessment methods have not been widely used because of the time and expense involved. However, there may be times when such an evaluation is needed. Often this need is identified when an individual presents him/herself to the physician for medical help with a health problem. Although a physician may perform an initial assessment, a person with advanced training in nutrition is needed to adequately assess history and pinpoint ongoing problems. A complete nutritional assessment should include a patient's health history, some assessment of socioeconomic status, a list of current and past medications, current dietary supplements, and a dietary history. Some blood and urine biochemical measurements can also be made if warranted. The evaluation should include measurement of height, weight, midarm circumference, waist-to-hip ratio, and fatfold (skinfold) thickness. A thorough assessment includes an examination of the whole body, and the individual should be examined for signs associated with particular nutrient deficiencies as listed in Table 5.2.

Table 5.2 Physical Signs of Malnutrition

Area of Body Examined	Common Signs of Malnutrition	Deficiency/Abnormality
Appearance in general	Significant overweight or underweight	Energy imbalance
	Apathetic or hyperirritable	Protein
	Loss or slowness of ankle or knee reflexes; pitting edema.	
Eyes	Paleness, dryness, redness or pigmentation of membranes (conjunctiva)	Vitamin A, riboflavin
	Foamy patches or conjunctiva (Bitot's spots)	Iron B_{12}, folate, copper
	Dullness, softness, or vascularization of the cornea	Excess, Wilson's disease
	Redness or fissures on eyelids	Hypercholesterolemia
Face	Rash, seborrhea, pallor	Riboflavin, iron, folate, B_{12}
Gums	Receded, "spongy" and bleeding; swelling of the gingiva	Vitamin C
Hair	Dullness; may be brittle and easily plucked without pain	Protein
	Sometimes lighter in color than normal (depigmentation may be bandlike when hair is held up to a source of light)	
Lips	Swollen, red, corners cracked (cheilosis)	Riboflavin
Muscles	Wasting and flabbiness of muscle; bleeding into muscle	Protein, iron, folate, B_{12}
Nails	Brittle and ridged nails; spooning	Protein, iron
Heart	Racing heartbeat (over 100 beats per minute)	
	Enlargement	Selenium
	Failure	Thiamin
	Abnormal rhythm	Magnesium, potassium, calcium
Organs	Palpable enlargement of liver or spleen	Alcohol abuse
	Ascites	Protein
Skeleton	Softening, swelling, or distorted shapes of bones and joints	Vitamins C and D
Skin	Roughness (follicular hyperkeratosis), dryness, or flakiness	Protein
	Irregular pigmentation, black-and-blue marks, lesions	Niacin
	Symmetrical, reddened lesions, rash, edema	Protein
	Looseness of skin (lack of subcutaneous fat)	Energy
	Flakiness, peeling, dry	Protein, zinc
Teeth	Caries, mottled or darkened areas of enamel	Fluoride excess
Tongue	Atrophy of papillae (the tongue is smooth) or hypertrophy of papillae	B_{12}, folate, riboflavin
	Swollen, scarlet, magenta (purple colored), or raw tongue	
	Irregularly shaped and distributed white patches	Iron

The most common reasons for office visits that may require nutritional intervention are problems related to hypertension, diabetes mellitus, degenerative joint disease, heart disease, pregnancy care, infant and child care, adolescent care, and obesity. Nutritional status assessment may also be a part of a general medical examination. The patient's medical and family history, the physical examination, and appropriate laboratory assessments can then be used to assess nutritional status. These can then be compared to nationally collected averages for these same measurements. One such widely known study is the NHANES (National Health and Nutrition Examination Survey). These surveys are conducted at regular intervals by the Centers for Disease Control and Prevention. Their methodology is available should the examination warrant such use. As a result of medical nutrition evaluation, patients may be categorized as normal, malnourished, or at risk of malnourishment. Malnourishment can include both over- and underconsumption of needed nutrients.

Nutritional Assessment

The patient who is starved, or who has a malabsorption problem, or who has hepatic, pancreatic, or renal disease, trauma, sepsis, cancer, or who requires critical care should be given special attention with regard to nutritional status assessment and subsequent nutritional therapy. A registered dietitian is an invaluable resource in assessing dietary intake by dietary recall, prospective food records, and food frequency questionnaires. The clinician (either physician or dietitian) needs to ask about the use of dietary supplements (vitamins, minerals, and others). Vitamin/mineral supplements are often used to optimize nutritional health and forestall disease development. Over-the-counter remedies and herbal remedies are also often used and are marketed with little restriction with respect to their efficacy or active ingredient content. Often patients do not report the use of such supplements and over-the-counter remedies. This can set the stage for deleterious interactions with respect to prescribed drugs, or further problems in the management of a particular disease state. Toxic adverse interactions between herbals and medications or foods can occur, and patients need to be informed about these potential problems.

While serious nutritional deficiencies have largely disappeared in affluent countries, they still exist, especially in patients who have other predisposing conditions. One such condition is alcoholism. If possible (some alcoholics are not willing to seek nutrition support), that condition should be addressed and nutritional support provided. The special needs of menstruating women are another of these special circumstances. The regular loss of menstrual fluids means that women are at risk of anemia and nutritional supplements may be needed to address their potential deficiencies of iron, copper, and some of the B vitamins. The postmenopausal woman is at risk of calcium loss from her bones and this too can be addressed from the nutritional and activity point of view as well as pharmacologically. Vegetarianism could be a concern if the patient is unaware of the need to ingest sufficient vitamin B_{12} and balanced protein. The special nutrient needs of pregnant and lactating women should also be a special consideration. Meeting the periconceptual (the period preceding conception) need for folic acid is a related special circumstance. In some women, especially those with a high folacin requirement, an inadequate intake of folacin prior to conception and in the early phase of embryogenesis could result in neural tube defects in the unborn child. Neural tube defects include spina bifida, hydrocephaly, and malformations of the neural system.

Gender differences need to be recognized with respect to body size, body composition, and metabolic/hormonal differences. All of these can impact nutritional status. Last, with increasing age and the effects of age on nutrient need, there should be concern about the nutritional status of the elderly. A number of instances of diseases common in the elder population have nutrition components. Conditions such as type 2 diabetes, obesity, vascular disease, dementia, and osteoporosis all have nutrition components. Intervention strategies instituted in middle life could be instrumental in delaying the development and onset of these degenerative diseases. Patients who cannot (e.g., because they are in a coma or have a broken jaw) or will not eat (anorexia) should be evaluated for possible enteral or parenteral nutrition support. Enteral support is the provision of nutrients via a feeding tube, while parenteral support is the provision of nutrients via a deep vein catheter.

Laboratory Tests

Laboratory tests can assist in the nutritional assessment and diagnosis of people at risk for malnutrition. Table 5.3 provides a list of such tests and the uses of these results. Since blood is a carrier tissue to and from organs, its content can be informative. Types of blood work may include a complete blood count (CBC), blood chemistry panels (glucose, electrolytes, minerals, lipids, indices of renal and hepatic function), and tests of blood coagulation as well as enzymes. Values from healthy adult individuals are shown in Chapter 1 (see Tables 1.3, 1.4, and 1.5).

Hemoglobin levels will show the presence of anemia that may be vitamin specific or mineral related and can indicate chronic disease. The red cell size and hemoglobin content and concentration can provide clues to liver disease, alcoholism, and specific nutrient deficiencies. While serum albumin is not a sensitive indicator of protein status, it does provide a clue. Low levels may indicate a limiting amount of substrate for hepatic protein synthesis. However, non-nutritional factors may be responsible for hypoalbuminemia such as expanded extracellular fluid, accelerated protein breakdown, and impaired renal and hepatic function. Albumin levels may be unreliable indicators of protein status in the postoperative or acutely injured patient. Some enzyme tests are indicators of nutritional cofactor status; for example, alkaline phosphatase for zinc and aminotransferase for vitamin B_6.

Malnutrition may also result from too much of a particular nutrient, as is the case when a person overdoses on fat-soluble vitamins (hypervitaminosis A or D) or consumes

Table 5.3 Laboratory Tests Useful in Clinical Nutritional Assessment

Test	Index for
Hemoglobin, hematocrit, red and white cell counts and differential (calculate total lymphocyte count)	Anemia, protein status
Urea, creatinine, glucose, sodium, potassium, chloride, CO_2	Renal function, diabetes, acid-base balance
Cholesterol, triglycerides, lipoproteins	Lipid disorders
Total protein, albumin, uric acid	Renal/hepatic function
Calcium, phosphate, magnesium, bilirubin, alkaline phosphatase	Skeletal disorders
Aminotransferases, iron, ferritin	Anemia, iron status
Transferrin, transthyretin, retinol binding protein	Iron status
Prothrombin time, partial prothrombin time	Vitamin K status

an excess of energy-rich food and stores the excess energy as fat (obesity). Drug/nutrient interactions can occur and perturb homeostasis. In some circumstances, these interactions may be deleterious. Some may be common; for example, the interaction of asthma medications with components of grapefruit juice. In this instance, both the asthma medications and components of the grapefruit juice use the same detoxification reactions in the liver. Because of competition for these detoxification reactions, the asthma medications are not detoxified as rapidly as normal and last much longer than expected. If the person with asthma consumes a lot of grapefruit juice (e.g., a quart of grapefruit juice at one time), a food–medication reaction could occur. If this food consumption pattern is not recognized and the dosing schedule not altered to accommodate the problem, the end result could be death. The expedient procedure would be to inform the patient of this potential interaction and either greatly reduce or eliminate grapefruit juice from the diet and/or adjust the medication schedule.

Case Study 5.1: Elise Complains of Trouble Driving at Night

Elise is a 67-year-old woman who visited her eye doctor because she had trouble driving at night. She thought she needed new glasses but that was not the case. Her visual acuity had not changed. What had changed was her self-imposed fat-free, milk-free diet. She used to enjoy salads and vegetables and a good steak. But she had been reading the health food literature and was concerned that her former diet was not good for her. She now consumes lots of cereal grains, and tubers, believing that the fat in her diet was not good for her. She also believed that the chemicals used to grow fruits and vegetables were harmful, so she eliminated them from her diet. She did, however, take a B vitamin supplement pill every morning. The problem she described was being unable to see the road after she passed an oncoming vehicle. This disturbed her and she was sure she would have an accident if she did not get some help.

Her ophthalmologist tested her for dark adaptation and light adaptation. She definitely had a problem adjusting to differences in light intensity.

Problem Analysis and Resolution

   1. What was Elise's problem?

   2. What caused it?

   3. What remedies would you suggest?

Case Study 5.2: Uncle John Is an Alcoholic

Uncle John is 43 years old. He has always been rather lean but lately he has lost some weight. He looks downright skinny. Uncle John is fun to visit, full of lots of funny stories, and very convivial. He seldom is without a bottle of beer in his hand. He really loves his beer and the guys at work drink about the same amount. He does not think he is an alcoholic! In a given day he might consume a six-pack of 12-oz bottles of beer and he feels that his friends do likewise. Sometimes he will snack on pretzels or potato chips to go along with the beer and occasionally he will have a hamburger with some fries. He says his appetite is poor. He seldom wants anything to eat, preferring to drink his beer.

Lately, Uncle John has noticed some scaliness on his arms and also some other skin changes. He seems more tired than usual and his face seems paler than it used to be. He was always an outside guy. He loved to watch sports and cheer for his favorite team. Now he is somewhat apathetic and listless.

Problem Analysis and Resolution

1. What is John's problem?

2. What remedy do you suggest and how can you implement this remedy?

3. What do you think will be the probable outcome for John if he does not accept the remedy offered?

Case Study 5.3: Little Lizzie Has Scurvy

Lizzie is 2 years old. She has begun to walk but has a funny skeleton. Her mother has noticed that the ends of her ribs have little knobs on them. Lizzie has her baby teeth, but her gums seem to bleed a lot and she is far more fussy than she used to be. When placed on her back in her bed, she spreads her legs with her little knees out.

Her mom was concerned so she brought Lizzie to the well-baby clinic at her local hospital. The doctors were dismayed because they realized that Lizzie's problem was scurvy. They promptly treated her with vitamin C and instructed Lizzie's mom to give her little girl fresh orange juice every morning. Thinking that the problem was fixed (the gums were healing and Lizzie's fussiness went away), they discharged Lizzie. Her mom took her home but a couple of weeks later she was back at the hospital with the same symptoms. The doctors were so frustrated. They asked Lizzie's mom if she had followed their instructions about giving Lizzie orange juice every day. "Oh yes," Lizzie's mom said. "I ran down to the corner store every morning and got Lizzie a fresh bottle of orange pop!"

Problem Analysis and Resolution

1. What is the problem here?

2. Lizzie's mom thought she was doing the right thing but she was not. Why?

3. What do you think needs to be done to remedy the situation?

chapter 6

How Is Food Used?

How Do We Get the Nutrients in the Food into Our Bodies?

Most people do not eat to consume nutrients. They consume food as part of their daily lifestyle choices. These foods must be broken down into absorbable components through the processes of digestion and absorption provided by the gastrointestinal system. This system consists of the mouth (oral cavity containing teeth, tongue, and salivary glands) esophagus, stomach (including the parietal cells and other cells that produce and release enzymes and other fluids necessary for digestion), the small intestine (including the cells that produce and release enzymes and those cells that produce and release hormones), large intestine, rectum, and anus. Some people would also include the liver and the duct connecting it to the gallbladder as well as the bile duct connecting the gallbladder to the small intestine. Bile, produced by the liver and stored in the gallbladder, is needed for the emulsification of food lipid and also serves as a conduit for the recirculation of several minerals as well as cholesterol. Another important accessory organ is the pancreas. This organ has both exocrine and endocrine functions.

Retrieval of nutrients from consumed food is a two-part process: digestion and absorption. Once food is consumed, digestion begins. Digestion can proceed only when the large particles of food are made smaller through chewing. As the food is chewed, it is mixed with saliva, which contains α-amylase and lingual lipase. These enzymes start the digestion of carbohydrate and lipid, respectively. The salivary α-amylase is denatured in the stomach as the food is mixed and acidified with the gastric hydrochloric acid. The lipase is acid stable and continues to work in the stomach.

Absorption

Absorption occurs after the food components are digested into their absorbable units. It occurs via the cells lining the gastrointestinal tract (enterocytes) by one of three mechanisms: active transport, facilitated diffusion, and passive diffusion. Active transport is a process that moves a substance against a concentration gradient. It requires energy (usually as ATP) and a nutrient carrier. Many carriers are specific for specific nutrients; some are not. Some carriers will transport several similar compounds. Many of the essential nutrients are actively transported. The exceptions are some of the micronutrients and the essential fatty acids. The minerals are absorbed either by passive diffusion or by a carrier-mediated transport mechanism (facilitated diffusion). Passive diffusion refers to the movement of a substance across the cell membrane so as to equalize its concentration on both sides of the membrane. This process applies to water, some electrolytes, some small sugars, and some nonessential amino acids. It does not apply to large molecules such as starch or protein. Essential fatty acids diffuse across the lipid portions of the enterocyte membranes. Facilitated diffusion is the movement of substances against a concentration gradient; it usually requires a carrier but may not require energy. A number of essential minerals are absorbed using this mechanism.

Protein Digestion

Protein digestion begins in the stomach. There, the food is acidified with the gastric hydrochloric acid produced and released by the parietal cells of the stomach. Sometimes these cells can release the acid in the absence of a food stimulus. This excess acid release can cause problems because the acid can destroy the protective mucus layer that coats the stomach. The hydrochloric acid serves several functions: It acidifies the ingested food, killing potential pathogenic organisms; it serves to denature the food proteins, thus making them more vulnerable to attack by pepsin, an endopeptidase; and it releases lipid from lipid-protein complexes.

As the food is mixed with the gastric acid and the gastric peptidases it becomes a slurry called *chyme*. Chyme passes to the duodenum of the small intestine where the amino acids in the acidic chyme stimulate the release (from the endocrine cells of the small intestine) of pancreazymin (also called *cholecystokinin*). This is a hormone that signals the exocrine pancreas to release pancreatic juice into the duodenum and bile from the gallbladder. The low pH of the chyme also stimulates the release of secretin, which in turn stimulates the exocrine pancreas to release bicarbonate and water. The bicarbonate works to neutralize the acidic chyme. This neutralization optimizes the environment for the duodenal enzymes needed for the digestion of the food ingredients.

Proteins are attacked by the proteases pepsin, parapepsin I, and parapepsin II of the gastric juice as well as by peptidases in the small intestine. It is begun in the stomach and finished in the small intestine. The proteins in the ingested food must be hydrolyzed into their component amino acids, dipeptides, and tripeptides prior to absorption. This is accomplished through a series of enzymes that target specific amino acid linkages as their point of action. These enzymes are summarized in Table 6.1. The protein hydrolases, called peptidases, fall into two categories. Those that attack internal peptide bonds and liberate large peptide fragments for subsequent attack by other enzymes are called the *endopeptidases*. Those that attack the terminal peptide bonds and liberate single amino acids from the protein structure are called *exopeptidases*. The exopeptidases are further subdivided according to whether they attack at the carboxy (-COOH) end of the amino acid chain

Table 6.1 Protein Digestive Enzymes and Their Target Linkages

Enzyme	Source	Target
Pepsin	Stomach	Peptide bonds involving the aromatic amino acids
Trypsin	Small intestine	Peptide bonds involving arginine and lysine
Chymo	Small intestine	Peptide bonds involving tyrosine, tryptophan, phenylalanine, trypsin, methionine, and leucine
Elastase	Small intestine	Peptide bonds involving alanine, serine, and glycine
Carboxy	Small intestine	Peptide bonds involving valine, leucine, isoleucine, peptidease A, alanine
Carboxy	Small intestine	Peptide bonds involving lysine and arginine peptidase B
Endo-	Cells of brush	Di- and tripeptides that enter the brush border of peptidase border the absorptive cells
Aminopeptidase	Cells of brush	Di- and tripeptides that enter the brush border of peptidase border the absorptive cells
Dipeptidase	Cells of brush	Di- and tripeptides that enter the brush border of peptidase border the absorptive cells

Table 6.2 Carriers for Amino Acids

Carriers	Amino Acids Carried
1	Serine, threonine, alanine
2	Phenylalanine, tyrosine, methionine, valine, leucine, isoleucine
3	Proline, hydroxyproline
4	Taurine, β alanine
5	Lysine, arginine, cysteine-cysteine
6	Aspartic and glutamic acids

(carboxypeptidases) or the amino ($-NH_2$) end of the chain (aminopeptidases). The initial attack on an intact protein is catalyzed by endopeptidases, and the final digestive action is catalyzed by the exopeptidases. The final products of digestion are free amino acids and some di- and tripeptides that are absorbed by the intestinal epithelial cells.

Amino Acid Absorption

Although single amino acids are liberated in the intestinal contents, there is insufficient power in the enzymes of the pancreatic juice to render all of the amino acids singly for absorption. The brush border of the absorptive cell therefore not only absorbs single amino acids but also di- and tripeptides. In the process of absorbing these small peptides, it hydrolyzes them to their amino acid constituents. There is little evidence that peptides enter the blood stream. There are specific transport systems for each group of functionally similar amino acids, di- and tripeptides. These carriers are listed in Table 6.2.

Most of the biologically important L-amino acids are transported by an active carrier system against a concentration gradient. This active transport involves the intracellular potassium ion and the extracellular sodium ion. As the amino acid is carried into the enterocyte, sodium also enters in exchange for potassium. This sodium must be returned (in exchange for potassium) to the extracellular medium. This return uses the sodium-potassium ATP pump. In several instances, the carrier is a shared carrier. That is, the carrier will transport more than one amino acid. Such is the case with the neutral amino acids and those with short or polar side chains (serine, threonine, and alanine). The mechanism whereby these carriers participate in amino acid absorption is similar to that described for glucose uptake.

Carbohydrate Digestion

As the food is chewed, it is mixed with saliva, which contains α-amylase. This amylase begins the digestion of starch by attacking the internal α 1,4-glucosidic bonds. It will not attack the branch points having α 1,4- or α 1,6-glucosidic bonds; hence the salivary α-amylase will produce molecules of glucose, maltose, α-limit dextrin, and malto-triose. The α-amylase in saliva has an isozyme with the same function in the pancreatic juice. The salivary α-amylase is denatured in the stomach as the food is mixed and acidified with the gastric hydrochloric acid.

The disaccharides in the diet are hydrolyzed to their component monosaccharides. Lactose is hydrolyzed to glucose and galactose by lactase, sucrose is hydrolyzed to fructose and glucose, and maltose is hydrolyzed to two molecules of glucose. Table 6.3 lists these enzymes together with their substrates and products. One of these enzymes, lactase,

TABLE 6.3 Enzymes of Carbohydrate Digestion

Enzyme	Substrate	Products
α-Amylase	Starch, amylopectin, glycogen limit dextrins	Glucose, maltose, maltotriose
α-Glucosidase	Limit dextrin	Glucose
Lactase	Lactose	Galactose, glucose
Maltase	Maltose	Glucose
Sucrase	Sucrose	Glucose, fructose

declines in activity after weaning. This decline is regulated at the level of transcription by factors that include the cessation of milk consumption. The identity of these regulatory substances has not been fully elucidated. Because the majority of humans in the world are lactose intolerant at adulthood and because milk contains so many essential nutrients in addition to lactose, it would be useful to understand the regulation of lactase gene expression. If one could prevent the age-related decline in lactase activity, milk and milk products could be used by more people to improve their nutritional status. Therapy for lactose-intolerant individuals consists simply of restricting lactose intake. There is a lactose-free milk on the market that provides all the nutritive value of whole milk without lactose. Some individuals tolerate fermented products such as yogurt and cheese fairly well, while varying amounts of fresh milk induce the typical symptoms of gastrointestinal discomfort, diarrhea, and flatulence.

As mentioned, starch digestion begins in the mouth with salivary amylase. It pauses in the stomach as the stomach contents are acidified, but resumes when the chyme enters the duodenum and the pH is raised. The amylase of the pancreatic juice is the same as that of the saliva. It attacks the same bonds in the same locations and produces the same products: maltose, maltotriose, and the small polysaccharides (average of eight glucose molecules), the limit dextrins. The limit dextrins are further hydrolyzed by α-glucosidases on the surface of the small intestine luminal cells, the enterocytes. The carbohydrates whose bonds are not attacked by α-amylase or α-glucosidase, or the disaccharidases, maltase, lactase, or sucrase are then passed to the lower part of intestine where they are attacked by the enzymes of the intestinal flora. Most of the products of this digestion are used by the flora themselves; however, the microbial metabolic products may be of use. The flora can produce useful amounts of short-chain fatty acids and lactate, as well as methane gas, carbon dioxide, water, and hydrogen gas. The carbohydrates of legumes typify the substrates these flora use. Raffinose, which is used by the flora, is converted to an α-galactose 1→6 glucose 1→2 β- fructose, trehalose, and α-glucose 1→1 α-glucose. These carbohydrates are the typical substrates from legumes for these flora. The flora will also attack portions of the fibers and celluloses that are the structural elements of fruits and vegetables. Again, some useful metabolic products may be produced, but the bulk of these complex polysaccharides have undigestible β linkages and are largely untouched by the intestinal and flora enzymes. These undigested, unavailable carbohydrates serve very useful functions:

1. They provide bulk to the diet, which in turn helps to regulate the rate of food passage from mouth to anus.
2. They act as adsorbants of noxious or potentially noxious materials in the food.
3. They assist in the excretion of cholesterol and several minerals, thereby protecting the body from overload.

Carbohydrate Absorption

Once the monosaccharides are released through the action of the carbohydrate hydrolyzing enzymes of the enterocytes and the pancreatic juice, they are absorbed by one of several mechanisms. Glucose and galactose are absorbed by an active transport mechanism that is energy dependent, sodium dependent, and carrier mediated. This mechanism is termed *active transport* because glucose is transported against a concentration gradient. Because the transport is against a concentration gradient, energy is required to "push" glucose into the enterocyte. Glucose and galactose appear to compete for the same active transport system. They also compete for a secondary transporter, a sodium-independent transporter (the mobile glucose transporter, GLUT 2) found in the basolateral surface of the enterocyte membrane. The two transporters differ in molecular weight. The sodium-dependent transporter has a molecular weight of 75 k Da while the sodium-independent transporter weighs 57 k Da. This sodium-independent transporter is a member of a group of transporters called GLUT 1, 2, 3, or 4. Each of these transporters is specific to certain tissues. They are sometimes called *mobile glucose transporters* because when not in use they reside in the endoplasmic reticulum. Under the appropriate conditions they move from the endoplasmic reticulum to plasma membrane where they fuse with the plasma membrane and bind glucose. Upon binding, the transporter and its associated glucose is released from the membrane. Through this mechanism the glucose enters the intestinal absorptive cell.

Fructose is not absorbed via an energy-dependent active transport system but by facilitated diffusion. This process is independent of the sodium ion and is specific for fructose. Once in the enterocyte, it too is transported by a mobile carrier. In the enterocyte much of the absorbed fructose is metabolized such that little fructose can be found in the portal blood even if the animal is given an intraluminal infusion of this sugar. However, an infusion of sucrose will sometimes result in measurable blood levels of fructose. The reason this occurs may be due to the location of sucrase (the enzyme that catalyzes the hydrolysis of sucrose to fructose and glucose) on the enterocyte. Rather than extending out into the lumen as do the other disaccharidases that are anchored to the enterocyte by a glycoprotein, sucrase is more intimately anchored. The sucrose molecule then is closely embraced by the enzyme, which in turn facilitates both the hydrolysis of sucrose and the subsequent transport of its constituent monosaccharides. Thus, both monosaccharides enter the enterocyte simultaneously. Of the other monosaccharides present in the lumen, passive diffusion is the means for their entry into the enterocyte. Pentoses such as those found in plums or cherries, and other minor carbohydrates, will find their way into the system only to be passed out of the body via the urine if the carbohydrate is not used.

Lipid Digestion and Absorption

The digestion and absorption of the various food lipids involves the mouth, stomach, and intestine. The digestion of lipid is begun in the mouth with the mastication of food and the mixing of the food with the acid-stable lingual lipase. Later, the churning action of the stomach mixes the food particles with hydrochloric acid. These actions separate the lipid particles, exposing more surface area for enzyme action and emulsion formation. The changes in physical state are essential steps that precede absorption. The remaining lipid components of the diet are mixed with other diet ingredients by the churning action of the stomach. Little degradation of fat occurs in this organ except that catalyzed by lingual lipase, which originates from glands in the back of the mouth and under the tongue. This lipase is active in the acid environment of the stomach. However, because of the tendency of lipid to coalesce and form a separate phase, lingual lipase has limited opportunity to attack the triacylglycerols (the simple lipids in fats and oils). Those that are attacked release a single fatty acid, usually a short- or medium-chain one. The remaining diacylglycerol is subsequently hydrolyzed in the duodenum. In adults consuming a mixed diet, lingual lipase is relatively unimportant. However, in infants having an immature duodenal lipase, lingual lipase is quite important. In addition, this lipase has its greatest activity on the tria-cylglycerols commonly present in whole milk. Milk fat has more short- and medium-chain fatty acids than fats from other food sources. Although the action of lingual lipase is slow relative to lipases found in the duodenum, its action to release diacylglycerol and short- and medium-chain fatty acids serves another function: These fatty acids serve as surfactants. Surfactants spontaneously adsorb to the water–lipid interface, stabilizing emulsions as they form. Other dietary surfactants are the lecithins and the phospholipids. Altogether, these surfactants plus the churning action of the stomach produce an emulsion that is then expelled into the duodenum as chyme.

The chyme's entry into the duodenum stimulates the release of the gut hormones, secretin and cholecystokinin into the blood stream. Secretin stimulates pancreatic bicarbonate release. Cholecystokinin stimulates the gallbladder to contract and release bile. Bile salts serve as emulsifying agents and to further disperse the lipid droplets at the lipid–aqueous interface, facilitating the hydrolysis of the glycerides by the pancreatic lipases. The bile salts impart a negative charge to the lipids, which in turn attracts the pancreatic enzyme colipase.

Cholecystokinin also stimulates the exocrine pancreas to release pancreatic juice, which contains three lipases (lipase, lipid esterase, and colipase). These lipases act at the water–lipid interface of the emulsion particles. One lipase acts on the fatty acids esterified at positions 1 and 3 of the glycerol backbone, leaving a fatty acid esterified at carbon 2. This 2-monoacylglyceride can isomerize and the remaining fatty acid can move to carbon 1 or 3. The pancreatic juice contains another, less specific lipase (called a lipid esterase), which cleaves fatty acids from cholesterol esters, monoglycerides, or esters such as vitamin A ester. Its action requires the presence of the bile salts. The lipase that is specific for the ester linkage at carbons 1 and 3 of the triacylglycerols does not have a requirement for the bile salts and, in fact, is inhibited by them. The inhibition of pancreatic lipase by the bile salts is relieved by the third pancreatic enzyme, colipase.

Colipase is a small protein (mol. wt. 12,000 Da) that binds to both the water–lipid interface and to lipase, thereby anchoring and activating the lipase. The products of the lipase-catalyzed reaction, a reaction that favors the release of fatty acids having 10 or more carbons, are these fatty acids and mono-acylglyceride. The products of the lipid esterase-catalyzed reaction are cholesterol, vitamins, fatty acids, and glycerol. The phospholipids present in food are attacked by phospholipases specific to each of the phospholipids. The pancreatic juice contains these lipases as prephospholipases, which are activated by the enzyme trypsin.

As mentioned, the release of bile from the gallbladder is essential to the digestion of dietary fat. Bile contains the bile acids, cholic acid and chenodeoxycholic acid. These are biological detergents or emulsifying agents. At physiological pH, these acids are present as anions, so they are frequently referred to as bile salts. At pH values above the physiological range, they form aggregates with the fats at concentrations above 2–5 mM. These aggregates are called *micelles*. The micelles are much smaller in size than the emulsified lipid droplets. Micelle sizes vary depending on the ratio of lipids to bile acids, but typically range from 40 to 600 Å.

Micelles are structured such that the hydrophobic portions (triacylglycererols, cholesterol esters, etc.) are toward the center of the structure, while the hydrophilic portions (phospholipids, short-chain fatty acids, bile salts) surround this center. The micelles contain many different lipids. Mixed micelles have a disc-like shape wherein the lipids form a bilayer and the bile acids occupy edge positions, rendering the edge of the disc hydrophilic. During the process of lipase and esterase digestion of the lipids in the chyme, the water-insoluble lipids are rendered soluble and transferred from the lipid emulsion of the chyme to the micelle. In turn, these micelles transfer the products of digestion (free fatty acids, glycerol, cholesterol, etc.) from the intestinal lumen to the surface of the epithelial cells, where absorption takes place. The micellar fluid layer next to this cell surface is homogenous, yet the products of lipid digestion are presented to the cell surface and, by passive diffusion, these products are transported into the absorptive cell. Thus, the degree to which dietary lipid, once digested, is absorbed depends largely on the amount of lipid to be absorbed relative to the amount of bile acid available to make the micelle. This, in turn, is dependent on the rate of bile acid synthesis by the liver and bile release by the gallbladder. People who have had their gallbladder removed still have their bile acids. Instead of stockpiling them in the gallbladder to be released upon the cholecystokinin signal, surgeons simply remove the gallbladder and make a direct connection between the liver and the duodenum. Once the fat has been absorbed, the bile acids pass on through the intestine, where they are either reabsorbed or conjugated and excreted in the feces.

The primary bile acids, cholic and chenodeoxycholic acids, are produced from cholesterol by the liver. They are secreted into the intestine, where the intestinal flora convert these acids to their conjugated forms by dehydroxylating carbon 7. Further metabolism occurs at the far end of the intestinal tract where lithocholate is sulfated. While the dehydroxylated acids can be reabsorbed and sent back to the liver via the portal blood, the sulfated lithocholate is not. It appears in the feces. All four of the bile acids, the primary and dehydroxylated forms, are recirculated via the enterohepatic system so that very little of the bile acid is lost. It has been estimated that the bile acid lost in the feces (~0.8 g/day) equals that newly synthesized by the liver so that the total pool remains between 3 and 5 g. The amount secreted per day is on the order of 16–70 g. Since the pool size is only 3–5 g, this means that these acids are recirculated as often as 14 times a day.

The function of the bile acids is thus quite similar to that of enzymes. Neither is "used up" by the processes they participate in and facilitate. In the instance of fat absorption, the bile acids facilitate the formation of micelles, which, in turn, facilitate the uptake of the dietary fatty acids, monoglycerides, sterols, phospholipids, and other fat-soluble nutrients by the enterocyte of the small intestine. Not only do these bile acids recirculate, but so too does cholesterol. Gallstones develop when the resecreted material is supersaturated with cholesterol, and this cholesterol-laden bile is stored in the gallbladder. With time, the cholesterol precipitates out, providing a crystalline structure for the stone. Since the bile also contains a variety of minerals, these minerals form salts with the bile acids and are deposited within and around the cholesterol matrix. Eventually these stones irritate the lining of the gallbladder or may lodge themselves in the duct connecting the bladder to the duodenum. When this happens, the bladder becomes inflamed, the duct may be blocked, and the patient becomes unable to tolerate food. In some cases, treatment consists of reducing the irritation and inflammation through drugs, but often the patient has the gallbladder and its offending stones removed. This surgery is called a cholecystectomy.

In this surgery the common bile duct is connected directly to the small intestine after the gallbladder is removed.

Virtually all of the fatty acids, as part of the mono-, di-, and triacylglycerides, and glycerol are absorbed by the enterocyte. Only 30–40% of the dietary cholesterol is absorbed. The percent cholesterol absorbed depends on a number of factors, including the fiber content of the diet, the gut passage time, and the total amount of cholesterol present for absorption. At higher intake levels, less is absorbed, and vice versa at lower intake levels. Compared with fatty acids and the acylglycerides, the rate of cholesterol absorption is very slow. It is estimated that the half-life of cholesterol in the enterocyte is ~12 hours. With high fiber intakes, less cholesterol is absorbed because the fiber acts as an adsorbent, reducing cholesterol availability. The different fibers vary in their adsorptive capacity with respect to cholesterol. Cellulose and lignens are good adsorbants of cholesterol, while transit through the intestine can be hastened by cellulose and hemicellulose. Pectins and gums increase transit time, yet they lower serum cholesterol levels by creating a gel-like consistency of the chyme, rendering the cholesterol in the chyme less available for absorption. High-fiber diets reduce gut passage time, which in turn results in less time for cholesterol absorption.

The fate of the absorbed fatty acids depends on chain length. Those fatty acids having 10 or fewer carbons are quickly passed into the portal blood stream without further modification. They are carried to the liver bound to albumin in concentrations varying between 0.1 and 2.0 meq/mL. Those fatty acids remaining are bound to a fatty acid–binding protein and transported through the cytosol to the endoplasmic reticulum, whereupon they are converted to their CoA derivatives and re-esterified to glycerol or residual monoacylglycerides to reform triacylglycerides. These reformed triacylglycerides adhere to phospholipids and fat-transporting proteins that are members of the lipoprotein family of proteins. This relatively large lipid–protein complex migrates to the Golgi complex in the basolateral basement membrane of the enterocyte. The lipid-rich vesicles fuse with the Golgi surface membrane, whereupon the lipid–protein complex is exocytosed or secreted into the intercellular space, which in turn drains into the lymphatic system. The lymphatic system contributes these lipids to the circulation as the thoracic duct enters the jugular vein prior to its entry into the heart.

The remaining lipid components of the diet are mixed with other diet ingredients by the churning action of the stomach. Little degradation of fat occurs in this organ except that catalyzed by lingual lipase, which is thought to originate from glands in the back of the mouth and under the tongue. This lipase is active in the acid environment of the stomach. However, because of the tendency of lipid to coalesce and form a separate phase, lingual lipase has limited opportunity to attack the triacylglycerols. Those that are attacked release a single fatty acid, usually a short- or medium-chain one. The remaining diacylglycerol is subsequently hydrolyzed in the duodenum. In adults consuming a mixed diet, lingual lipase is relatively unimportant.

Vitamins and minerals are absorbed as separate entities. Some of the vitamins are absorbed via an active transport system, while others require a carrier and still others are absorbed passively. Many of the essential minerals are absorbed passively, but several require specific carriers.

Case Study 6.1: Steven Has a Belly Ache

Steven is a 45-year-old store manager who is complaining of a burning, gnawing pain, moderately severe, almost always in the epigastric region. The pain is absent when he wakes up in the morning but appears about midmorning. It is relieved by food but recurs 2 to 3 hours after a meal. This pain often wakes him up during the night. Endoscopic examination of his gastrointestinal tract showed normal stomach anatomy but craters and inflammation were observed in the duodenum. Gastric analysis demonstrated that the gastric juice pH fell to 1.9 with pentagastrin stimulation (6 ug/kg s.c.). Fasting serum gastrin levels were normal.

Problem Analysis and Resolution

Using your textbook and any other sources of information, answer the following questions:

1. Based on your understanding of the function of the gastrointestinal system, what do you think is the problem?

2. What is the significance of a pentagastrin stimulation test? (What is pentagastrin?) What is the significance of the fasting serum gastrin measurement?

3. Suggest some over-the-counter remedies to ease the symptoms. Why and how do these work?

4. Suggest some dietary alterations that may help get these symptoms under control. If the pain emanated from the stomach with acid reflux, would the management remain the same? What other diagnoses could be entertained?

Case Study 6.2: John Has a Pain

A college student, John, complained of pain, nausea with vomiting, and tenderness in the lower right quadrant. He had not been involved in any unusual physical activity. The pain was more of an ache at first but became worse as time went on. It hurt more when he moved or breathed deeply, coughed, or sneezed. After a couple of days, he developed a mild fever of 102.2°F, and moderate leucocytosis (11,500/cu mm) was found on blood workup. His right lower quadrant had pronounced tenderness at McBurney's point (one-third the distance between the anterior superior iliac spine and the umbilicus) upon examination. He exhibited pain on hyperextension of the thigh.

Problem Analysis and Resolution

1. What do you think is wrong with this guy (beyond a longing for the semester to end!)?

2. Describe in anatomical terms the location of the organ involved. Prepare a sketch of its location.

3. What is the cause of the fever, pain, and leukocytosis in this person?

4. If left untreated, what is the next clinical "outcome" for this student?

5. What is the usual treatment for this disorder? Will a dietary adjustment help this student?

Case Study 6.3: Emily's Baby

Emily and Dennis were delighted to welcome their second child, a daughter, into the world last September. As they soon discovered, there is a cloud to every silver lining. When baby Shasta was about a month old, Emily and Dennis began to notice a pattern in their routine for baby care. At the same time every day, Shasta would become very fussy. This fussiness usually began suddenly. Her legs were drawn up and her small belly appeared bloated. Although Shasta appeared to get some relief when she passed gas or a stool, most episodes ended when she had vomited a significant amount of stomach contents. Needless to say, she did not gain weight appropriately. Shasta is being breast fed and has yet to begin solid foods.

Problem Analysis and Resolution

Based on the story above, answer the following questions:

1. What is Shasta's problem?

2. Suggest a diet for Emily that may aid Shasta's problem.

3. Are there any potential health issues that Emily and Dennis may want to be watching for as relates to Shasta's diet during her growth years?

Case Study 6.4: Herbert Is on a Food Supplement Kick

Herbert has Type 1 diabetes mellitus. He is 40 years old and has had the disease for about 30 years. He has managed his glucose homeostasis very well but lately has developed an interest in the natural foods movement. He has immersed himself in their literature and has learned that vitamins and minerals are important to good health. As a diabetic he has always known that he must carefully manage what he eats so as to balance his food intake against the insulin he injects on a regular basis. But having achieved middle age, he has become very health conscious. He has begun taking a multivitamin supplement as well as several mineral supplements to boost his magnesium, calcium, iron, copper, and chromium intake. After a few days of beginning to consume all these supplements, he notices that he has diarrhea every midmorning. This is a real change in his usual pattern and the diarrhea has affected his glucose control.

Problem Analysis and Resolution

1. Explain what has happened.

2. What should Herbert do to change this situation?

Case Study 6.5: Herman Is Convinced He Has Heart Trouble

Herman is a 26-year-old business executive. He is mildly overweight with a large abdominal fat pad. Lately, he has been complaining of a dull pain behind the sternum. The pain is postprandial and intermittent. Many times it would disappear in a few minutes but sometimes it might last up to an hour. It was often associated with belching and was worse when lying down or after meals high in meat protein and fats. The pain was sometimes intense enough to radiate to the back, jaws, shoulders, and down the inner aspect of the arms. Herman was afraid it might be heart related because it seemed similar to what he had heard about heart disease. Herman decides finally to see his physician who orders several tests. His electrocardiogram was normal, with no indication of cardiovascular disease. Radiographic studies of his esophagus and stomach revealed a small portion of the stomach above the diaphragm. An endoscopic biopsy revealed mucosal inflammation. Esophageal manometry revealed decreased lower esophageal sphincter pressure. Esophageal pH monitoring showed lowered pH measurements particularly close to the esophageal side of the sphincter.

Problem Analysis and Resolution

Based on this case study, your textbook, and other outside sources, answer the following questions:

1. What is Herman's problem?

2. Why did Herman experience more pain when lying down? What mechanisms normally prevent this problem when (a) standing, (b) lying down, and (c) bending over?

3. What sort of dietary recommendations would you make to limit this problem?

4. Do you have suggestions for sleeping comfortably?

5. What sort of pharmaceutical remedies (can be natural or manufactured) would you suggest to limit the number of episodes?

6. What other remedies could you suggest for Herman?

We Are What We Inherit

Over the last 50 years, there has been a growing interest in the individuality of nutrient need and tolerance. We have learned that our genetic background can influence how much of each of the individual nutrients are needed by our bodies. Similarly, we have also learned that individuals differ in their optimal intakes of certain nutrients. For example, some people require far less vitamin A than do others; for some, what might be adequate vitamin A intake might be inadequate for others, and for a third group the same amount might border on toxic. The tolerable range is large, yet there can be instances where too much would elicit an adverse response. The daily recommended intakes (DRIs) contain safety factors such that if they are followed, the consumer should be adequately nourished and avoid toxicity.

Biochemical individuality has been known to exist for decades, and nutrition scientists have realized that the recommendations of nutrient intakes must allow for this. Hence the early intake recommendations were made such that nearly all people could avoid the consequences of deficiency if they followed these intake recommendations. Now, however, scientists have come to realize that some intake recommendations are inappropriate for some people. For example, the energy intake recommendation is very uncertain (there is no energy DRI) because if only a single energy intake was provided it might be too little for one individual while for another it would be too much and could result in excess fat storage. This is perhaps the most interesting example of how nutrients and genetic heritage interact to determine the nutrient needs of the individual. Other instances can be cited as well. However, before these instances are listed, it is important to consider how genes are expressed and how nutrients affect this expression.

Nutrition scientists have been interested not only in how nutrients affect gene expression but also how small differences in the base sequence of a given gene or in the factors that influence gene expression could affect the gene product and subsequent nutrient need or tolerance. Scientists have been especially interested in how specific nutrients function as promoters or suppressors of specific genes. This area of research is quite active.

What Is a Gene? What Is Our Genotype? What Is Our Phenotype? What Is the Difference between the Terms, Genotype and Phenotype?

DNA, found in the nucleus and mitochondria of cells, is a chain of bases (adenine, guanine, thymine, and cytosine) connected by phosphate groups and deoxyribose (a sugar). A gene is a specific segment of that chain. Altogether the chain is referred to as the *genome*. The human genome, in general, has been sequenced. That is, we know the order of the bases from start to finish of the DNA in the "average" human. We know that variation does occur in this sequence, yet the full implications of these variations are not known entirely. Despite the fact that human DNA has been sequenced, it has not been fully mapped. That is, we do not know the purpose of each gene within our chromosomes. We do not know where each gene is located on the DNA chain. We also do not fully understand how the expression of each of the genes is regulated. We know a lot about some of the genes but almost nothing about other genes. Many of the genes of importance to physiology, nutrition, and metabolism have been sequenced and identified but not all are known. There are some genes that influence the expression of other genes, while there are a few that produce gene products whose function is unknown. This is a *very* active and exciting research area.

The function of DNA is to provide the blueprint for all of the proteins that give a cell, tissue, organ, and individual its characteristic traits. As mentioned, DNA is composed of four bases: adenine, guanine, thymine, and cytosine. Species vary in the percent distribution of these nucleotide bases in their DNA. These bases are linked together by a condensation reaction to form the DNA chain in a process analogous to the condensation of amino acids that serve as the primary structure of a protein. The sequence of amino acids in each protein synthesized by the body is determined from a subunit of the DNA molecule known as the gene. A gene can have as few as 27 bases or as many as several thousand for the unique combination of amino acids that characterize every protein and peptide in the body. Each amino acid has a specific triplet of bases (its codon) that encode it. Some amino acids have more than one triplet. While only four bases are used for the DNA, the base triplets and sequences of these triplets provide a specific code for each protein and peptide in living systems. For any given gene the sequence of bases in that gene is the *genotype* of that individual for that particular gene. Thus, the sequence of bases in the gene provides the blueprint for the sequence of amino acids that compose the resultant gene product, whether it is a protein or a peptide. This in turn gives the cell, tissue, organ, or individual the traits that describe it, whether it is the color of the hair, the function of an organ, or the biochemical activity of the cell. This characteristic is then called the *phenotype* of the individual.

As mentioned above, variation in individuals can and does occur in the DNA sequence. If there is a difference in the sequence of the nucleotides within the DNA, there are four possible consequences. First, because several of the amino acids have several different codons (the triplet of bases that dictate a particular amino acid in the gene product or protein), there might be no difference at all in the amino acid sequence of the resultant protein. Second, if the base substitution occurs in a part of the DNA that is not used in the transcription of the RNA for a given protein, again, there would be no effect on the resultant protein. Third, if the base substitution occurs in the DNA that encodes a portion of the resultant protein that contributes nothing to the active site of the protein or to its structural form, then, again, the base substitution would have no effect on the resultant gene product. This can occur because several of the amino acids possess similar functional characteristics. Last, if the base substitution occurs such that the sequence of amino acids in the resultant protein is functionally different in the critical active portion of the resultant protein, then that protein might malfunction. These consequences are grouped into two groups: If the change results in an aberrant gene product (the protein it encodes), it is called a *mutation*. If the change has no effect on the gene product or its function, it is called a *polymorphism*. The term *polymorphism* is also used to describe variation in the amino acid sequence of proteins with identical functions. In these instances, there can be slight, but not major, differences in function or activity.

In some instances of DNA base substitutions, there are no outward effects of these substitutions on the resultant protein if that protein is of little consequence to the overall function of the body. For example, a mutation in the gene for the pentose metabolizing enzyme (NADP-linked xylitol dehydrogenase) needed to metabolize the pentoses in cherries and plums has little significance to the body. Seldom is it a problem. People who enjoy plums and cherries may excrete that pentose in the urine without realizing that it has not been metabolized normally. However, if the protein whose amino acid sequence has been changed is crucial to the normal functioning of the organism, then this change is serious indeed. For example, if the base substitution (mutation) occurs in the active site for the protein glucose 6-phosphatase, the final enzyme in the gluconeogenic sequence, then a serious disease (von Gierke's disease, Type I glycogen storage disease) results. This rare disease is characterized by intermittent and severe hypoglycemia and also results in an enlarged liver and other metabolic abnormalities that in turn result in a shortened life span of the affected person.

Mutations can occur spontaneously or may be induced by exposure to DNA-damaging materials or other adverse conditions. Subsequent generations of cells will then have this mutation in their DNA. If the mutation occurs during fertilization, during embryogenesis, or during fetal growth, the resultant individual could have a genetic disease or could have characteristics typical of that mutation. The mutation could result in a devastating condition if it occurred in a crucial portion of the DNA or it could be simply a variation from normal. As described above, base substitutions in the DNA or even base deletions/additions might result in a serious problem *or might not* depending on the nature of the change in base sequence of the DNA. If a mutation occurred in any of the chromosomes except the sex chromosomes, it is an autosomal mutation. If it occurred in either the X or Y chromosome, it is a sex-linked mutation. With respect to the variations in base sequence of DNA, the possibilities are endless. Thousands of genetic diseases due to variation in specific genes have been described. Some are very common and others are rare. It is the variation in DNA that contributes to the uniqueness of each individual, each tissue or organ, and each cell. Before we can discuss this endless variation, we must first understand how the process works.

How Do We Inherit Our Genotype and Phenotype?

As mentioned, the process of protein synthesis uses the sequence of bases in DNA as the blueprint for the sequence of amino acid in the protein. The DNA sequence of bases determines the unique properties of each cell type, since the properties that make cells unique are usually conferred by the proteins within them. Some of these proteins are the structural elements of the cell. Others are enzymes that catalyze specific reactions and processes that characterize the cell in question. Still other proteins confer a particular biochemical function on the cell.

During cell division, the nuclear DNA, as soon as its replication is completed, becomes highly condensed into distinct chromosomes of characteristic shapes. These chromosomes exist as pairs and are numbered. There are 46 chromosomes in the human. Included in this number are the sex chromosomes, the X and Y chromosomes. If the individual has one X and one Y, he is a male; if two Xs are present, she is a female. The chromosomes are the result of a mixing of the nuclear DNA of the egg and sperm. Approximately half of each pair comes from each parent. If identical codes for a given protein are inherited from each parent, the resultant progeny will be a *homozygote* for that gene and resultant protein. If nonidentical codes are inherited, the progeny will be a *heterozygote*. Within the heterozygote population, there may be certain codes that are *dominant*, the codes for eye color or hair color, for example. These are dominant traits and are expressed despite the fact that the individual has inherited two different codes for this trait. A code (and resultant protein) that is not expressed is a *recessive* trait. If by chance two identical recessive genes are present that encode a certain protein, the trait will be expressed. This is the basis for the genetic diseases of the *autosomal* recessive or dominant type. *Autosomal* means a mutation in any of the chromosomal DNA except that which is in the X or Y chromosome. A mutation of the DNA in this chromosome is called a *sex-linked* mutation. If it results in a disease, it is called *sex-linked genetic disease*. An example here is the expression of the trait for hemophilia. The hemophilia trait is carried on the X chromosome. Only males express the trait because they have only one X chromosome. Females have two X chromosomes and since the trait is a recessive one, their other X chromosome will dominate and they will not express the hemophilia trait. They will carry it and pass it on to their sons should that particular X be passed. There is a 50:50 chance that their sons will receive the mutated X chromosome at conception. Not all of their sons will have the trait and indeed only 50% of their daughters will receive the trait and pass it on to their progeny. There is another inheritance pattern based on the mitochondrial genome. Because this genome is primarily of maternal origin, certain of the characteristics of the OXPHOS system will be inherited via maternal inheritance. A number of mitochondrial mutations result in a number of degenerative diseases.

How Does Our Environment Shape the Phenotypic Expression of Our Genotype?

Gene–nutrient interactions can account for a wide variety of disease states. As already mentioned, genetic variation can explain why some nutrient intakes are too low for some people while being adequate for others. Some of the chronic diseases likewise have both a nutrition component and a genetic component. Diseases such as heart disease, diabetes mellitus, and obesity are in this category. Last, there are a number of genetic conditions that in turn can be managed by diet. One of the most common of these is lactose intolerance. About 75–80% of the adult population in the world today is lactose intolerant. That is, they cannot consume quantities of milk and some milk products without experiencing gastrointestinal distress.

Although many genetic signatures have been associated with specific diseases, not all people who have these genetic characteristics actually develop the associated disease. This suggests that one must not only have the genetic characteristic, but also provide the environment for the disease to flourish. A beautiful example of this was reported in the early 1960s. Newly arrived Yemenite Jews and Yemenite Jews who had resided in Israel for at least 20 years were compared with respect to diet, lifestyle, and the prevalence of type 2 diabetes. The newly arrived immigrants had very little diabetes, while the established Yemenite Jews had as much diabetes in their population as the Israeli Jewish populations from other parts of the world. The diets and lifestyles of these population groups were compared to a matched group of Arabs living in the same locations in Israel. The diets were not greatly different among the groups yet the disease was far more prevalent in the Jews than in the Arabs. Studies of the diet consumed by the Jews in Yemen versus that in Israel revealed that there were very few differences with one exception: In Yemen, very little refined carbohydrate was consumed. Sugar was not readily available, and what was available was very expensive. Once the Yemenites settled in Israel and adopted the Israeli diet with its abundance of refined carbohydrates, type 2 diabetes began to appear. It was suggested that the change in diabetes prevalence in the Yemenite group was due to an interaction between their genetic heritage and their increased consumption of refined carbohydrate. This report was the first to suggest such an interaction. Other nutrient–gene interactions have been suggested, and it has been difficult to determine which of these proposed interactions has merit. Through the study of a wide variety of families and population groups, more than 150 mutations have been reported that associate with diabetes mellitus, yet the presence of one or more of these mutations does not necessarily mean that the person will become a diabetic. Diabetologists have acknowledged that there are far more people with a diabetes genotype than with a diabetes phenotype. That many of the diabetes phenotypes take so many years to develop suggests that given the appropriate lifestyle choices the phenotype might never develop or might develop very rapidly, depending on these choices. In support of this argument, one has only to look at the numbers of new cases of diabetes in times of abundant food supplies and in times of food restriction. During World War II, when food was rationed (as was gasoline for automobiles), people ate less and were more active. During this period the number of new cases of type 2 diabetes fell. The number of new cases of type 1 diabetes (autoimmune diabetes or insulin-dependent diabetes) remained fairly constant. Because food was rationed and activity was increased due to the rationing of gasoline, fewer people had excess fat stores and this was probably a contributing factor to the decrease in diabetes development. When food and gasoline became abundant after the war, food intake again was unrestricted and people became more sedentary, and the prevalence of both diabetes and obesity rose.

Some forms of diabetes and obesity share a genotype that phenotypes as obesity and diabetes, called *diabesity*. As with the group of diseases called *diabetes*, obesity has a number of mutations that associate with it and, as mentioned, some of these mutations phenotype as obesity and diabetes that codevelop together. The expression of these genotypes depends largely on whether abundant food is available and consumed to make possible the phenotypic expression of the obesity and diabetes genotype. Several of these mutations affect food intake regulation and thus affect energy balance. If the brain does not receive an appropriate appetite-suppressing signal, then excess energy is consumed with the result of excess body fat stores. Excess fat stores, particularly in the adipocyte, interfere with the action of insulin in facilitating the entry of glucose into the cell. This is called *insulin resistance*. When this occurs, abnormal glucose metabolism (type 2 diabetes) develops. Individuals with excess fat stores can normalize their glucose metabolism if these stores are significantly reduced through food intake restriction and increased physical activity. However, not all instances of diabesity can be resolved in this way.

Even though we know that these chronic diseases have a genetic linkage, we are, at present, unable to identify individuals genetically before their disease develops. Here is where a good family medical history would be important. Individuals having close relatives with one or more of these diseases are much more likely to develop them than people without these diseases in their family. Knowing that these conditions are influenced by lifestyle choices, if susceptible individuals could be identified (even just knowing the family history), it should be possible to develop effective strategies to forestall disease development. It might not be possible to eliminate the problem, but it could delay its appearance appreciably.

Some obesity phenotypes might be very obvious while others are not. An example of the former is the synthesis of three related proteins important to energy balance regulation. These proteins are the uncoupling proteins 1, 2, and 3 (UCPs). The UCPs function to uncouple the synthesis of ATP from the synthesis of water in the mitochondrial compartment. If UCPs are present, the cell makes less ATP and releases more energy as heat (thermogenesis), thereby decreasing energetic efficiency. If one or more UCPs is absent or nonfunctional due to a mutation(s) in the codes for these proteins, the reverse occurs. More energy is trapped in the high-energy bond of ATP, and this energy is subsequently transferred to synthetic reactions that produce storage energy products: fats and glycogen. With a decrease in energy wastage by the mitochondria, excess fat accumulates. There is a very limited capacity to store glycogen. For whatever reason, the individual is unable to produce or release one or more of the UCPs, and fuel metabolism and energy balance are adversely affected. That individual may not be able to rapidly adjust to changes in environment such as a dramatic drop in environmental temperature. Here is an example of a nutrient–gene interaction that is part of a disease process—in this case, obesity. However, it is not a single nutrient but the overconsumption of all energy-containing nutrients—carbohydrates, fats, and proteins—that plays a role in obesity development.

With this mutation as well as with others that associate with obesity, if the individual does not have access to a plentiful food supply, the obesity phenotype might not develop. Some have argued that these genetic changes occurred many generations ago and that it was probably one that ensured survival under the adverse conditions of an intermittent food supply. Those people with the mutation(s) were far more able to survive periodic starvation than those people without this genetic change. In today's world there is an abundant food supply, and what was once a survival characteristic is now a liability. Obesity due to an overconsumption of food with subsequent efficient energy storage capacity is a leading risk factor for type 2 diabetes, heart disease, renal disease, and so forth.

There are numerous examples of specific nutrient effects on transcription. Some of these effects concern the transcription of genes that encode enzymes, or receptors or carriers that are important to the use of that nutrient. Many nutrients serve more than one function with respect to gene expression. Some influence both transcription and translation, while others serve to enhance the transcription of one gene while suppressing the transcription of another. Nutrient–gene interactions can result in either an increase or a decrease in a specific mRNA or a group of RNAs, yet there may be no increase in gene product or a measurable increase in gene product function. This speaks to the complicated nature of metabolic control.

Some nutrients affect translation. An example of an effect of a specific nutrient on translation is that of iron in the synthesis of ferritin. Iron storage in cells occurs through chelation to a protein called *ferritin*. This occurs at the outer aspect of the mitochondrial membrane. Ferritin synthesis is highly regulated by iron intake. In iron deficiency, the mRNA start site for ferritin translation is covered up by an iron-responsive protein. This protein binds the 3′UTR start codon and inhibits the movement of the 40s ribosome from the cap to the translation start site. When the diet contains sufficient iron and iron status is improved, the start site is uncovered and translation then proceeds. After translation is complete, the primary amino acid sequence is complete. The secondary and tertiary structure of the protein evolves via numerous interactions between amino acids via hydrogen bonding, disulfide bridges, and ionic bonds. The newly synthesized proteins can be further modified via post-translation reactions, and again nutrients can affect this process. Post-translational protein modification includes the association of various subunits of an enzyme or a carrier or a cell component. For example, the association of the four subunits that make up hemoglobin occurs after the initial synthesis of each of the subunits has occurred. Another example is the post-translational carboxylation of the proteins, osteocalcin and prothrombin. Osteocalcin and prothrombin each have glutamic acid-rich regions that when carboxylated allow the protein to bind significant amounts of calcium. Calcium binding is an essential feature of the functions of each of these proteins. The post-translational carboxylation of osteocalcin and prothrombin requires vitamin K. Should vitamin K be in short supply, this carboxylation will not occur (or will occur in only a limited way) and these proteins will not be able to bind calcium. Both must bind calcium in order to function. Hence vitamin K deficiency is characterized by prolonged blood clotting times (inadequate calcium binding by prothrombin) and poorly mineralized bone (inadequate calcium binding by osteocalcin).

Finally, even though we know that nutrients can affect gene expression and that many chronic diseases have a genetic linkage as well as a nutrient linkage, our technology for identifying individuals at risk for some of these conditions is in its infancy. At present, we can identify individuals only after their symptoms become apparent, not *before* their disease develops. Knowing that these conditions are influenced by lifestyle choices, if we could identify susceptible individuals it should be possible to develop effective strategies to forestall disease development. In the short term, it is not possible to change a genotype, but early identification might delay the phenotypic expression of that genotype. If that were possible, health outcomes would be notably affected. As can be seen, we are indeed what we inherit from our parents. However, what we inherit can be modified by our lifestyle choices. The following activity should help you understand how your personal health can be affected by what you have inherited vis-à-vis genetic tendencies to develop some diseases.

Learning Activity 7.1: Your Family Tree

Prepare a four-generation family tree showing all of your biological relatives. You will need to ask your family members to provide this information. When you make the tree, do not give names to your family members, to protect their privacy. Give each one a number. Begin numbering either with your generation or with your great grandparents' generation. It does not matter where you begin—number with respect to the generations. However, each generation should have its own first number. For example, you might start with your generation. You would be #1, your sister would be #2, and your brothers would be #3 and #4. Your parents would be #10 and #11; their brothers and sisters likewise, double digits. Be sure to keep the family lines separate. That is, do not put all your father's sisters and your mother's sisters together, but separate them by families. Your grandparents' numbers would be triple digits, and your great grandparents would have four digits. If you are adopted this might not apply to you, but you should go through the activity anyway. Do not include step relatives, that is, stepsisters, step-parents, and so on. Show yourself, your siblings, parents, aunts and uncles, grandparents, grandaunts and uncles, and your great grandparents, aunts, and uncles. With each individual show whether he/she is alive or dead by providing birth dates and death dates (if applicable). If dead, indicate cause of death as well as any chronic conditions he/she might have had before death. If alive, indicate the presence of all medical problems. There may be many. List them all. Indicate any congenital problems and any genetic problems. Once you have put this tree together, you will then look at it to determine whether there might be any significant trends that could have significance with respect to your medical future. For example, you might note whether there is a lot of type 2 diabetes mellitus or a lot of colon cancer. These are diseases that have strong genetic linkages, but they are diseases that can be avoided or postponed with appropriate intervention.

After you have considered and completed your family tree, think about the following case studies. They have been written to help you understand situations where inheritance as well as lifestyle choices can impact the health and wellbeing of the individual.

Case Study 7.1: An African Adventure

John and Mary are excited by their upcoming trip to Africa. In preparation for their trip, they visit their doctor, who pronounces them fit and healthy enough for their adventure. Their doctor prescribes prophylactic doses of quinine since they will be visiting an area of Africa where malaria is endemic. Mary tolerates the quinine very well but after a week John begins to complain of feeling tired. Two weeks after beginning to take the quinine John is really under the weather and is feeling poorly. The two return to the doctor, who orders a full-scale clinical examination of John. His blood work shows that the red cell count has fallen from 5.8 to 3.9 million cells/cubic millimeter. There is evidence of extensive hemolysis. By the time the lab results are in, John is close to collapse and the doctor admits him into the hospital for care.

Problem Analysis and Resolution

1. What do you think has happened to John? How could he go downhill so quickly?

2. Explain how John but not Mary has a problem with the quinine.

3. Describe the genetic problem that is involved.

Case Study 7.2: BoBo Hates Milk; It Gives Him a Tummy Ache

BoBo, his nickname, is a delightful 4-year-old boy. He is developing normally and is growing adequately. His mom, however, is concerned that he is not eating right. She has read that young growing children should consume milk because it is an excellent source of calcium for strong bones and teeth. It is a good source of easily digested protein and contains essential vitamins and minerals. Every time she gives BoBo a glass of milk he avoids drinking it. He plays at the table and eventually manages to tip the glass over and spill the milk on the floor. His mom gets upset and cleans up the mess but doesn't think about BoBo's behavior as an avoidance mechanism. Finally, she forces BoBo to drink the milk. Within an hour BoBo has a tummy ache. He cries, draws his little legs up to his tummy, and clearly is very uncomfortable. After a couple of hours he expels some gas and has a bit of diarrhea and then is back to his sunny self.

Problem Analysis and Resolution

1. Based on the above story, what do you think is the problem?

2. What do you think BoBo's mom should do?

Case Study 7.3: Sylvia, Raymond, and Reginald Have a Fat Mother with Type 2 Diabetes

Sylvia, Raymond, and Reginald are siblings in their 30s. They live in close proximity to each other, frequently joining their mother for Sunday dinner and other family events. Their mother is an excellent cook who always encouraged her children to clean their plates of very generous portions. Sylvia was the first to notice that their mom was getting heavier than she had been. In fact, Sylvia tried to get her mother to join her in an exercise club. Mom did not want to do this because she was tired enough as it was and did not think she had what it took to go to an exercise session three to four times a week. Sylvia was dedicated to her exercise program. She even signed up for additional activities and decided to begin to train for marathon running. It was hard at first but eventually she became fit enough to run her first race. Mom was on the sidelines cheering her on until she collapsed into a chair. Sylvia became alarmed. She got her mom to an urgent care center as soon as she could. Mom was transported to the local hospital. Her blood work revealed a glucose level of over 500 mg/dL. She had indeed gained a lot of weight and her entry weight was 375 pounds. She was not very tall so this meant that she was very fat indeed. Over the years Sylvia had become used to seeing her mother always with a glass of iced tea or some beverage close at hand. She had also noticed how frequently her mom had to use the bathroom. Unfortunately Sylvia did not connect the dots. She did not realize, until mom collapsed, that her mom had become diabetic. The hospital stay put it all together. Mom had type 2 diabetes. The doctor first started mom on metformin to see if oral medication would get the glucose level down. This did not work so he then prescribed insulin injections, and mom was instructed on how to inject herself and how to check her blood glucose. A diabetes educator worked with her to help her develop a food plan that she liked. The clinicians also began a mild exercise program with mom's consent. Sylvia agreed to help mom adjust to this new lifestyle and mom got her glucose under control. Sylvia began to look at her brothers. Although Raymond was 35 and Reginald was 39, she noticed that they were both becoming increasingly fatter and sedentary. Where they used to play touch football on Sunday afternoons at family gatherings, now they were content to watch a game on TV. Sylvia worried that they were going to follow in mom's footsteps.

Problem Analysis and Resolution

1. Does Sylvia have something to worry about?

2. Based on the above story, what do you think is the problem with this family?

3. How likely is it that all three siblings will follow in their mother's footsteps?

4. What are the consequences for these siblings if this happens?

5. What strategies would you suggest and implement for this family?

6. Will the outcome for all three siblings be the same?

chapter 8

Pets and People

People have lived with animals almost as long as there has been life on earth. Animals have been companions and helpmates. They have provided food for their human caregivers as well as materials for shelter and for clothing. Anthropologists have found evidence for these associations that date back to prehistoric times. A wide variety of creatures have associated with humans. Included are fish, horses, dogs, cats, goats, cows, sheep, turtles, frogs, and reptiles. Some of these are merely pets that fascinate their human owners, while others assist their humans in their daily lives. Dogs, for example, in addition to being faithful companions, help their humans hunt, herd cows, sheep, and goats, lead the blind, and help the handicapped with their daily lives. Cows, sheep, goats, and pigs provide food as well as other materials for clothing and homes. Horses provide transportation and haulage. A variety of pets have been demonstrated to create stress-reducing environments for people. Pets can soothe humans, aiding in relaxation and helping these people maintain a relaxed lifestyle. In addition, studies of animals other than humans help scientists understand how the human body works. Comparisons of humans with other mammals and with nonmammals allow for the study of species differences and similarities.

Even though humans have had long associations with other species, the associations have not been trouble free. Some animal diseases can be transmitted to humans. These diseases are called *zoonotic diseases*. A zoonotic disease is one in which the infecting organism has its normal habitat in a nonhuman species but can produce disease in humans. Humans become infected by contact with contaminated animal products. Mad cow disease and AIDS are examples of zoonotic diseases. Zoonotic diseases are also diseases that can be transmitted from one species to another, for example, the transmission of rabies to a dog when bitten by a rabid possum. Other diseases develop when humans come in contact with animals that serve as vectors for pathogens that afflict humans; for example, bird flu and cow pox. Sanitation (both human cleanliness and the cleanliness of the animals they keep) and appropriate food handling techniques can prevent some of these problems, while immunization can prevent other problems. Some people develop allergies to the animals that they live with. Other people develop allergies to the foods these creatures provide. Still others become allergic to the clothing made from the hair or wool of these creatures. Why do some people have these problems while others do not? A lot of this can be explained by genetically controlled differences in the immune system. People with strong, specific antibody responses to foreign substances such as pathogens or allergens remain unaffected. However, many people either react slowly or overreact to immune challenges from foreign materials.

How the Immune System Works

The immune system is a complex system involving a cascade-like series of reactions culminating in the destruction of a foreign substance or pathogen. These substances are called *antigens*. The antigen may enter the body in many ways: It could be inhaled, it could penetrate the skin, or it could be swallowed with food or beverage. Regardless of how it enters the body, it elicits an immune response. First, the antigen is recognized as a foreign substance. Next, macrophages, dendritic cells, and B-cells bind the antigen. The B-cells are lymphocytes produced by the bone marrow. The antigen is processed and then presented to the T-cells, another type of white blood cell. These are cells produced by the thymus gland. Antigens are bound by the B-cells and presented to the T-cells. On the surfaces of these antigen-presenting cells are specific proteins that allow these cells to target specific types of antigens. These proteins are the major histocompatibility proteins or MHC proteins. There are two types of MHC proteins that are recognized by the T-cells when these proteins are bound to antigens. This recognition is due to specific receptors (immunoglobulins) on their surfaces. The T-cells themselves are divided into two groups: CD4s and CD8s. This division is based on the types of accessory factors (adhesion molecules) that are needed for the binding of the T-cell to the antigen-MHC complex on the presenting cell. The binding of the T-cell to the antigen-MHC complex then activates the T-cell, and this activation results in the release of one or more cytokines. This cascade of reactions is shown in Figure 8.1.

An antigen is either engulfed by a macrophage and destroyed or bound by macrophages, dendritic cells, and B-cells and presented to T-cells. This activates the T-cell, and it produces helper T-cells and killer (cytotoxic) T-cells. The helper cells help the B-cell to produce antibodies (shown as Ys). Altogether the cytotoxic T-cells, the macrophages, and the antibodies join forces, and the antigen is destroyed. Also involved are some cytokines. Cytokines are peptides that serve as signaling molecules. The cytokines ensure communication between the various components of the immune system as well as to cells outside of the system, for example, endothelial cells, bone marrow cells, and fibroblasts. The cytokines are used to control local and systemic immune and inflammatory events. More than 30 of these compounds have been identified. Included are the tumor necrosis factors (TNF), interleukins (IL), interferons (IFN), and colony stimulation factors. These cytokines can have local actions (paracrine) or distant actions (autocrine) and because of this, they may be regarded as hormones. The macrophage-derived cytocrines (IL-1, IL-6, and TNFα), for example, exert actions on distant organs.

Antigen-activated T-cells are termed T-helper cells because they "help" to mediate the cellular and humoral immune responses. Type 1 helper T-cells produce IL-2, IFNτ and

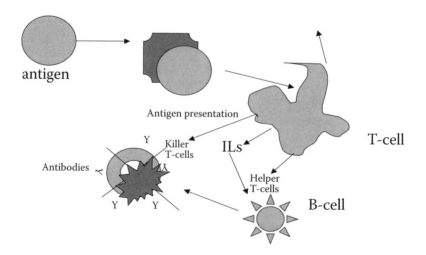

Figure 8.1 How the immune system works.

TNF-β, whereas type 2 helper cells produce IL-4, IL-5, and IL-10. The macrophages release IL-10 and IL-12. IL-12 signals cell-mediated immunity, whereas IL-10 acts as an anti-inflammatory agent. It does this by inhibiting the production of the other interleukins. The activity of the helper T-cells can be suppressed by a different T-cell known as a *suppressor T-cell*. The suppressor T-cell serves as a "brake" on the immune process such that an over-activation does not occur.

There is a third type of T-cell: the killer cell, or the cytotoxic cell. This cell is the executioner that surrounds and annihilates the infected or foreign cell. The antigen–antibody reaction has immobilized the pathogen or the foreign protein and this immobilization is followed by phagocytosis, during which the killer cell engulfs the foreign material and kills it. In contrast to the T-cells that adhere to the antigen (cell-mediated immunity) as already described and illustrated in Figure 8.1, the B-cells produce antibodies that adhere to the surface of foreign cells or to foreign proteins. Thus the foreign cell or protein is rendered inactive by the antigen–antibody reaction. Collectively, then, the antibody–antigen reaction and the phagocytosis exercised by the macrophages and the killer T-cells work together to ensure that the foreign cell or protein is rendered harmless.

Some of the B-cells are the so-called memory cells. They produce soluble immunoglobulin antibodies that remain in the blood plasma after the body is rid of the initial infection. These memory cells maintain a high degree of recognition specificity. Once exposed to a specific antigen they will produce this antibody with a high degree of fidelity. This is the basis of the immunization procedures used in infants to protect them from some of the communicable diseases. When challenged with an antigen, the memory cell is transformed into short-lived plasma cells. Plasma cells are protein factories that can produce –2000 antibody proteins/second during their brief (5–7 days) lifespan.

Antibodies

Antibody structures have been well studied. Most of the antibody molecules are similar in structure. However, antibodies differ in the tips of their Y-shaped structures. At the end of each of the points of the Y are different amino acid sequences that are dictated by the antigen to which it binds. It is estimated that there are ~10^{20} antibody molecules in each individual. Some of these will cross-react to closely related antigens. The antibodies are divided into five classes based on their respective roles in the immune system: IgG, IgA, IgE, IgM, and IgD. The IgG class is the main class of antibodies that are elicited by immunization or exposure to environmental pathogens. IgA antibodies are thought to be those present in bodily excretions (saliva, mucus, colostrum, etc.). These are the antibodies present in mother's milk and passed to the suckling infant to provide passive immunity to that infant. They are also the antibodies present in gamma globulin, which is frequently given to people exposed to a potentially dangerous pathogen so as to ward off serious disease. In each of these instances the effects of these passively acquired immune system components is of short duration (~3 months) but sufficient to allow the individual to develop his/her own antibodies to specific antigens.

IgE is involved in allergic reactions. These antibodies stimulate the release of histamines and other materials that in turn are responsible for the symptoms of an allergic reaction. Often, people with airborne allergies can take an antihistamine drug to inhibit histamine release, thereby suppressing the allergic response. IgM is an initial recognition molecule and is thought to trigger the IgG response. IgD antibodies function as antigen receptors on B-lymphocytes prior to antigen exposure. The latter two classes may have other functions as well, but these are not well described.

Types of Diseases of the Immune System

All disease states have a cause. Not all diseases are due to an infective agent. Some are actually diseases caused by the immune system itself. These are divided into four types. There are several types of diseases involving the immune system (Table 8.1). Type I disease is the group of diseases known as *allergies*. In this situation, the body manufactures IgE antibodies that attach to basophiles in the blood and mast cells in tissues. If an antigen is encountered, IgE stimulates the release of powerful mediators of inflammation (histamines, leukotrienes, and eicosanoids). These mediators produce the symptoms of an allergic reaction to an environmental antigen such as a pollen or a specific food ingredient. If the patient makes too much IgE in response to exposure to an antigen, a runny nose, watering eyes, or other symptoms of allergy will appear. In some cases (~10%) the allergic response is so overwhelming that the individual requires medical assistance. Without assistance the person might die. Instances of a bee sting or exposure to peanut protein eliciting anaphylactic shock are examples of such reactions. Injections of epinephrine are needed immediately to ward off the anaphylactic shock that follows exposure.

Type II immune disease is autoimmune disease. *Autoimmune disease* is a generic term covering a disease state in which the body develops antibodies to its own proteins and then proceeds to destroy cells containing these proteins. For some unknown reason the body loses its ability to recognize self-proteins and instead recognizes these as foreign. It then develops antibodies not only to these self-proteins but to other closely related proteins. Some of these may be cell surface proteins that are similar to dietary proteins. Thus when a person's blood is tested for the presence of antibodies to specific food proteins, there is a cross-reaction and it appears as though these food proteins are in the circulation. This is very unlikely. Nonetheless, because of the loss in specificity of antigen recognition, antibodies that react with food proteins can be found in these individuals. In autoimmune diabetes mellitus, the pancreatic β cells are destroyed, leading to an absolute insulin deficiency. The destruction is mediated by the T-cells producing antibodies of the IgG class in the immune system. There is an inflammation of the islet cells (insulitis) and these cells will contain both CD4 and CD8 T-cells, B-cells, macrophages, and killer T-cells. Antibodies to a variety of antigens can be found in the circulating blood of people with autoimmune type 1 diabetes. These include antibodies to glutamic acid decarboxylase, insulin, the insulin receptor, carboxypeptidase H, and c-peptide. Most of these antibodies are to cell surface proteins, thus supporting the mechanism of β cell destruction by antibodies that target this particular cell type. Autoimmune disease is not unique to the β cell. It can strike a number of different cell types. For example, the autoimmune disease psoriasis occurs when the immune system destroys the epidermal cells. Thyroid cells can

Table 8.1 Types of Immune Diseases

Type	Problem	Example
I	Excess IgE production	Food allergies, environmental allergies
II	Loss of antigen recognition specificity; inadequate suppressor T-cells,	Autoimmune diabetes, psoriasis, rheumatoid arthritis
III	Leaky cell membranes allowing soluble cell components to act as antigens	Lupus, adverse response to some drugs, glomerulonephritis, arthritis, rash, pleurisy
IV	Loss of helper cells	Tuberculosis; AIDS

be destroyed in the disease thyroiditis, which in turn develops as Hashimoto's disease (hypothyroidism). The connective tissue and the cells in the material around the joints can be destroyed through autoimmunity involving both IgM and IgG in rheumatoid arthritis. Swollen and painful joints, particularly in the hands and lower extremities, characterize this arthritis. All of these diseases can be retarded with the use of immunosuppressants such as cyclosporin. Studies of children newly diagnosed with autoimmune diabetes have shown that the time course of their disease can be retarded with the use of low doses of cyclosporin. Cyclosporin is one of the drugs used to prevent rejection of transplanted organs but when used in lower doses can affect the time course of autoimmune disease. There are other immunosuppressants that may be useful as well. Methotrexate, for example, is used in the treatment of rheumatoid arthritis.

Type III immune disease arises when antibodies to soluble cell components such as DNA or some cytoplasmic protein are formed. It is thought that this disease is due to a "leaky" plasma membrane. Such a membrane allows soluble cell constituents to "leak" out of the cell and in so doing these constituents are recognized by the immune system as "foreign." Systemic lupus erythematosus is an example of this type of immune disease. It develops when the body manufactures antibodies to DNA. The immunopathology of this type of immune disease involves a reaction to a cell-soluble antigen. That is, the antibodies are produced to materials found inside the cell and the cells are destroyed.

There is a fourth group of immune diseases that are T-cell mediated. They can be autoimmune diseases but usually the autoimmunity is a secondary effect. For example, in tuberculosis most of the destruction of the air sacs due to cavity formation (destruction of the epithelial cells lining the air sacs in the lungs) is T-cell mediated, not bacterium mediated. Similarly, in acute viral hepatitis, most of the liver destruction occurs via killer T-cells attacking the virus but incidentally killing the liver cell as well. In another example, the AIDS virus HIV-1 infects helper and induced T-cells because its envelope glycoprotein, gp 120, binds to the CD4 on their surface. Once inside the cell, the virus uses the enzyme reverse transcriptase to copy its RNA into the cells' DNA. It then becomes latent only to be reactivated when the T-cell responds to an antigen. Ultimately this results in a loss of helper cells, and the infected individual loses the response to infective agents. In other words, the patient's cells are destroyed not by the HIV-1 virus but by the body's failed immune system.

As can be seen, there are a number of mechanisms involved in reactions to foreign substances, be they pathogens, allergens, or self-proteins. All involve the immune system, which includes B-cells, T-cells, signaling molecules, and cytokines. All involve the development of antibodies, but the similarities end there. Whereas in the allergic reaction or the reaction to a pathogen the body is responding to a very specific allergen (antigen), in autoimmunity the reverse is true. The body loses its ability to recognize specific antigens and instead responds to a group of similar antigens. In autoimmune disease this loss of specificity means that the immune system has lost its ability to distinguish exogenous proteins or antigens from self-proteins or antigens. Proteins normally found in the plasma membrane are recognized as antigens rather than as normal cell constituents. Through this loss of recognition specificity, the body then develops antibodies that react to not only exogenous proteins, but also to its own cell proteins and, in so doing, destroys the cells of which these proteins are a part. The following case studies have been prepared to help with the understanding of the immune system as it relates to the body's response to different immunological challenges. An additional case study is presented that will allow for the exploration of species differences in the physiology of the respiratory system.

Case Study 8.1: The Horse with the Flying Tail

Reagan was the horse everyone wanted to own. She was tall and well built and moved beautifully. She had a kind and willing personality and she loved her owner, who tried to give her the sun, the moon, and the stars. One thing her owner couldn't give her was a rodent-free barn to live in. As Reagan got older, she began to have more and more problems with sores on the bottoms of her legs. Her owner worked diligently to medicate and care for her legs and she seemed to be healing. However, a few months after the onset of the skin problems, Reagan began to keep one eye shut all the time. At first, her owner thought it was insects, since the summer weather had been warm and dry. Her owner couldn't blame her for keeping her eye shut since her owner was also having trouble focusing her eyes. Regular bathing and care did not seem to help Reagan so her vet was called. Reagan was treated with several different medications but was finally referred to a large animal treatment clinic at the local veterinary teaching hospital. There she was diagnosed with recurrent equine uveitis and placed on cyclosporin treatment.

Problem Analysis and Resolution

1. What is uveitis? Trace the course of Reagan's problem.

2. Could her living conditions have contributed to her development of uveitis?

3. Is it possible that her owner also got this disease?

Case Study 8.2: Chuck Has a Parakeet

Chuck is 8 years old and he loves his pet Chirpy, a parakeet. The parakeet imitates Chuck's singing and the two spend a lot of time together. Chuck takes Chirpy out of his cage and the bird sits on Chuck's shoulder. Chuck is very responsible and feeds his bird as well as cleans up the bottom of the cage on a regular basis. One day the parakeet seemed listless and no longer responded to Chuck's company. The next day the parakeet was lying on the floor of the cage, dead. Chuck was very unhappy. A week later, Chuck developed a runny nose, fever, headache, and lung congestion. No one in the household had a cold or any other disease. None of his friends had been sick, either. When taken to the doctor Chuck was prescribed some tetracycline but this seemed to take a long time to help. After a week Chuck seemed to get better, but it took nearly 3 weeks before he was back to his normal cheerful self.

Problem Analysis and Resolution

1. What do you think caused this little boy to get sick?

2. Why were antibiotics only slowly effective? Describe the agent being attacked by the antibiotic.

3. What kind of an immune response was involved? How did it work?

Case Study 8.3: Elizabeth Has a Dog Problem

Elizabeth's family has a large retriever as a pet. The family has become very fond of this animal. However, over the years Elizabeth has noticed that whenever she pets the dog, brushes him, or cleans his doggy bed, her eyes water, she gets a severe sinus headache, and her nose runs. She loves the dog but when she is away visiting her cousins, who have no pets in the house, her sinuses clear up, her eyes are no longer red and watery, and her headache disappears. She visits the cousins as often as she can to get some relief from this congestion.

Problem Analysis and Resolution

1. What do you think is Elizabeth's problem?

2. What can she do about it?

3. What strategies would you suggest she employ to avoid the problem?

Case Study 8.4: Betty Changes Allegiances

When Betty finishes college, she congratulates herself on becoming a free, independent woman who is in charge of her own life. She has a diploma and some job skills, a car, a place to live that is not mom and dad's, and bills. Although going out on her own is exciting, Betty has elected to keep some things from her old home. One of those things is her cat, Oscar, which, unlike the family dog, never elicited an allergic reaction. However, since Betty is young and broke, she must make some choices. One of the choices she makes is to buy the least expensive dry food for her cat. Since fast food (mice) is in short supply, Oscar eats the food and looks woeful. After a few months, he looks more than woeful. In fact, he develops a dry, scaly skin, and is always scratching. This produces a cloud of cat dander in the air of Betty's living space. Most of Betty's old allergic problems begin to return.

Problem Analysis and Resolution

1. What caused Oscar's original problem? How could it be solved?

2. Will this help Betty?

Case Study 8.5: Julia Is Thin

Julia is 28 years old. She is 5′6″ tall and weighs 103 pounds. She has had intermittent bouts of diarrhea, painful abdominal cramping, bloating, and a lot of flatus. She is tired all the time and her boss has reprimanded her for not completing her assigned work in a timely manner. Julia has a hard time keeping warm. She wears a sweater all the time even in the middle of the summer. Julia is quite discouraged and her mom suggests that she go to the doctor for a complete physical. Her blood workup reveals hemoglobin level at 8.2 g/dL, red cell count 3.8 million/mm^3, hematocrit 30%, ferritin 18 μg/ml, red cell folate 200 nmol/L, and B$_{12}$ 100 pg/L. The doctor orders a bone scan using DEXA and this reveals a measure of osteoporosis. The doctor then suggests that Julia fill out a food intake form. A dietitian evaluates the results and cannot find any indication that Julia is inadequately nourished. The doctor scratches his head for an appropriate diagnosis when suddenly, while Julia is in his office, she has to make a rush visit to the lady's room. For some reason, Julia had failed to mention her gastrointestinal problems. Now it becomes obvious that an endoscopy and biopsy of the intestine is needed. The endoscopy examination reveals that the villi of the small intestine are shortened and in some areas are flattened and inflamed. Now the doctor needs to know why this occurred, so he orders a scraping of the lining of the intestine as well as an immune system workup. The results of these tests show an increase in MHC class II molecules, and these molecules do not have a normal shape. Further tests show that these molecules react to the proteins in wheat, rye, and barley but not to corn or rice.

Problem Analysis and Resolution

1. Based on your reading and your Internet searches, what do you think is Julia's problem? Why is she tired all the time? Why does she need a sweater when everyone else is going sleeveless?

2. Why is her diarrhea intermittent?

3. How do you explain her clinical results?

4. What strategies would you suggest that will make Julia's life more comfortable?

chapter 9

Food and Health

Food Safety

Food-borne illness has probably affected everyone at one time or another. It could occur when traveling or at home. It could occur at family picnics, grange hall dinners, or church bazaars. It can affect both wealthy and poor. It does not discriminate. Fast food restaurants or high-class, white tablecloth restaurants, or even Grandma might serve food that is contaminated with pathogens that could cause anything from a minor discomfort to a major life-threatening illness. This is a major concern for consumers, restaurants, and food producers, distributors, and processors. Last year, the CDC reported 76 million food-borne illnesses; 325,000 affected people were hospitalized and 5000 died. During the last decade, several new food-borne pathogens have been discovered and foods that traditionally have been considered safe have been implicated. With the increased globalization of the food supply, the origin of the contamination may be difficult to determine. Added to this is the increased consumer demand for preservative-free foods, convenience foods, and ready-to-eat meals. Outbreaks of food-borne illness are costly not only to the consumer in terms of healthcare costs and time lost from work, but to the food producer as well. The food producer could suffer a major economic loss that in turn could put the business into economic jeopardy. The pathogens listed in Table 9.1 vary in the foods that carry them. In general, foods that are undercooked, poorly refrigerated, or improperly washed prior to consumption are likely vectors for the pathogens.

Food-Borne Pathogens

Bacteria

Bacteria are a major agent of microbial food-borne illnesses. Food may be contaminated via contact with feces, soil, polluted water, or unsanitary food handlers. Bacterial food-borne illnesses can be classified into food-borne infections resulting from ingestion of foods containing viable cells of bacterial pathogens and food-borne intoxications that result from the consumption of foods containing preformed toxins produced by toxigenic bacteria but not by the bacteria themselves. The various bacterial pathogens associated with food-borne diseases are listed in Table 9.1.

Food-borne illness typically requires a very short incubation time and symptoms of gastrointestinal distress are common to most of the illnesses. The sources of contamination vary. *Escherichia coli*, a Gram-negative bacteria, can be found in humans and cattle, as these species serve as reservoirs of the bacterium. However, outbreaks of food-borne illness due to this bacterium have been associated with the consumption of raw or undercooked beef, unpasteurized milk, apple juice, lettuce, alfalfa sprouts, and contaminated water. The usual contaminate is fecal material, since *E. coli* is resident in the intestinal tracts of humans and cattle. Sometimes meat is contaminated at the slaughterhouse when the intestinal contents are spilled onto the carcass at slaughter. Other ways food may be

Table 9.1 Pathogens That Can Cause Food-Borne Illness

Pathogen	Symptoms or Disease
Bacteria	
Enterohemorrhagic *Escherichia coli*	Hemorrhagic colitis, hemolytic uremic syndrome, and thrombocytopenic purpura
Salmonella (several species*)*	Prolonged and spiking fever, abdominal pain, diarrhea, and headache
Campylobacter species	Enteritis: abdominal cramps, diarrhea (*C. jejuni* and *C. coli*), headache, and fever lasting up to 4 days
Shigella (several species)	Diarrhea containing bloody mucus, which lasts 1 to 2 weeks
Yersinia enterocolitica	Acute enteritis, enterocolitis, mesenteric lymphadenitis, terminal ileitis
Vibrio (3 species)	Gastroenteritis
(*V. parahaemolyticus*; *V. vulnificus*; and *V. cholera*)	When *V. cholera* is the agent, severe diarrhea, fever, dehydration; potentially fatal if fluids and electrolytes are not replaced
Aeromonas hydrophila	Watery diarrhea, mild fever
Listeria monocytogenes	Listerosis; potentially fatal to the elderly, pregnant women, and fetuses
Staphylococcus aureus	Nausea, vomiting, diarrhea, and abdominal pain
Clostridium botulinum	Paralysis due to a neurotoxin
Clostridium perfringens (5 types)	Produces an enterotoxin that causes diarrhea
Bacillus cereus	Induces vomiting, nausea, and watery stools
Brucella (6 species)	Causes brucellosis
Helicobacter pylori	Causes stomach ulcers that are responsive to antibiotics
Viruses	
Hepatitis A virus	Nausea, abdominal pain, jaundice, fever
Norwalk-like viruses	Nausea, vomiting, diarrhea
Rotavirus	Fever, vomiting, diarrhea
Avian influenza virus	Systemic infections, fever
Molds	
Aspergillus species	Can produce aflatoxins that may cause cancer
Penicillium species	Can produce a toxin that causes disease
Fusarium graminearum	Produces a toxin that causes anorexia, nausea, vomiting, diarrhea, dizziness, convulsions
Parasites	
Giardia lamblia (G. intestinalis)	Cramps, nausea, diarrhea, weight loss, anorexia
Entamoeba histolytica	Abdominal pain, fever, vomiting, diarrhea, bloody stool
Trichinella spiralis	2 phases: (1) abdominal pain, fever, vomiting, diarrhea; (2) edema, myalgia, difficult breathing, thirst, profuse sweating, chills, weakness, prostration
Cryptosporidium parvum	Profuse watery diarrhea, abdominal pain, nausea, vomiting
Cyclospora cayetanesis	Watery diarrhea, nausea, vomiting, myalgia, weight loss
Toxoplasma gondii	Fever, headache, muscle pain, lymph node swelling, abortion in pregnant women
Anisakis species (threadworms)	Epigastric pain, nausea, vomiting
Taenia species (tapeworms)	Nausea, epigastric pain, nervousness, insomnia, anorexia, weight loss, digestive disturbances, weakness, dizziness
Diphyllobothrium latum	Nausea, epigastric pain, diarrhea, pernicious anemia (large tapeworm)

contaminated include the use of raw, unprocessed fecal material as fertilizer on field crops, and contamination from food handlers who have not washed their hands after toileting.

Salmonella contamination likewise can be found in raw or undercooked meat. In addition, eggs, raw milk, raw shellfish, and other undercooked foods can be vectors for *salmonella*, *Shigella* contamination, and *Camplobacterium* contamination. These can also be found in raw or undercooked poultry, pork, and beef, as well as unpasteurized milk (*Campylobacter*) and other raw foods contaminated by unclean water. Uncooked or undercooked pork is the principal vector for *Yersinia* contamination. The various *Vibrio* contaminants are usually the result of the use of raw fecal material as fertilizer on food crops. These food crops must be thoroughly washed and rinsed in a chlorine solution to rid the food of this contamination. One of the *Vibrio* species caused widespread cholera in the countries in the Middle East in the 1970s. Contamination of the local water supply also accounts for outbreaks of *Vibrio*-related illness. Shellfish contaminated with these species are likely contaminated when the surface water containing raw sewage enters the shellfish growing beds. The shellfish are not affected but the consumers of this shellfish are. *Listeria* contamination of raw milk, soft cheeses, paté, and ready-to-eat meat products has been documented. Listerosis is serious in pregnant women as it can cause the death of the unborn child.

Staphylococcus aureus has been found in ham, chicken, and egg salads and also cream-filled pastries, mainly due to unsanitary practices of the food handlers and also due to unsafe storage conditions of the prepared foods. Salads must be kept cold to prevent the growth of this pathogen in these prepared foods. *Clostridium* contamination is serious indeed. The *Clostridium botulinum* produces a neurotoxin that causes life-threatening paralysis. It is a contaminant of meat, some home-canned vegetables, and sometimes honey. The contamination can be destroyed if the food is subjected to long periods of heat. Acid (below pH 4.6) also destroys the pathogen. *Bacillus cereus* is widespread in nature and can be found in cereals, rice, potatoes, cooked meat, milk and dairy products, spices, and dried foods such as raisins. The illness this pathogen causes is of short duration, lasting 24 to 36 hours, and can be prevented by keeping cooked foods hot (above 60°C) and cold foods cold (below 5°C).

Brucella is a contaminant of raw milk. Cows testing positive for this organism are culled out of a milk cow herd to reduce the possibility of milk contamination. Raw milk and products made from the raw milk are the sources of this pathogen in the human food supply. Last, *Helicobacter pylori* has recently been discovered to contaminate foods via contaminated water. Humans consuming food or beverages contaminated with this pathogen develop gastric ulcers that are cured by the administration of antibiotics. The ulcers are painful yet treatable if recognized as a food-borne illness.

Viruses

Viral contaminants of food can cause serious illness such as hepatitis A. Unfortunately most antibiotics are not very helpful in the treatment of the illness that follows exposure to such viruses. All of the known viral contaminants produce similar symptoms of nausea, vomiting, fever, diarrhea, and other symptoms typical of the specific virus involved. The source of the virus is contaminated water and unsanitary conditions in the preparation of the food. Consuming raw shellfish grown in sewage-contaminated water has been implicated in many cases of hepatitis A as well as in norovirus-caused illness. We do not know precisely how the avian flu or bovine spongiform encephalopathy viruses are transmitted.

Eukaryotic Contaminants (Molds and Parasites)

The molds that contaminate the human food supply are usually found in grain products. The molds produce aflatoxins, which are thought to cause some forms of cancer and in other instances may cause miscarriages (spontaneous abortion) in pregnant women.

Most of the parasitic diseases come about through the consumption of sewage-contaminated water. Food plants watered with this contaminated water can also serve as vectors for the parasites. Some of the parasites (*Trichinella*, *Anasakis*, *Taenia*, and *Diphyllobothrium*) enter as larval cysts in meat. If consumed undercooked, these larva mature in the intestinal tract and can migrate to other parts of the body. The long tapeworm and the round worms usually stay in the intestinal tract, but the *Trichinella* (trichinosis) and *Anasaki* migrate. Some round worms have been found to migrate in severely infected individuals.

Recognition

The symptoms of food-borne illness are quite similar regardless of the pathogen involved. Nausea and vomiting are the first symptoms that the body is trying to get rid of the pathogen. The diarrhea that follows is another attempt by the body to rid itself of the pathogen. After these symptoms mitigate, the disease state segregates depending on the source of contamination and how much of the contaminated food has been consumed. If the illness is of short duration, the individual may not seek medical help and the incident will not be recognized as a problem by the Public Health Service. If large numbers of people report symptoms to their physicians or public health workers, the CDC may be called in to find the source of the contamination and the identity of the pathogen. They will then try to correct it if possible. Good detective work is essential to define and identify the culprit pathogen and institute corrective measures to limit further contamination and future illnesses.

Prevention

The prevention of food-borne illness is the most important strategy. Cleanliness in food production and handling all along the chain from grower to consumer is of paramount importance. Avoiding fecal contamination of the food in the fields and in the processing centers is the key to this prevention. Isolating and identifying microbiological contaminants is important, as is the development of processing strategies that kill contaminants before the food reaches the consumer. As described, there are a variety of microbial contaminants. Other hazards include contamination of the food with nonfood components such as heavy metals or as happened in China with the introduction of melamine into food products.

Case Study 9.1: Traveler's Tummy

Cancun, here we come! Spring break is coming and, oh, are we going to have fun! Stan, Ed, and Billy decide to drive from Alabama to Mexico and vacation at the resorts in Cancun. Being on student budgets, they decided to travel together in Billy's car. They decided to eat as cheaply as possible and perhaps sleep on the beach once they got there. They started off on Friday morning after their last class and were on the road for several hours when they became hungry. They stopped for a quick bite at a roadside farm store that sold sandwiches and beverages out of a water-cooled chiller. The food was not very chilled, but, oh well, it was food and these guys wanted some food. They ate and then back on the road they went. They had been on the road only a few hours and had not even reached Texas! After the lunch break, with Billy still driving, they reached the edge of Mississippi and were heading into Louisiana. It was about 4 p.m. when Stan started to feel "funny." An hour later, he told his buddies, "I think we need to stop. I'm gonna throw up." They stopped and Stan lost his lunch. A few minutes later Ed also admitted to not feeling well and they stopped again for him to lose his lunch. Billy was then the driver with two nauseous passengers. A couple of hours later, Stan told Billy they had to stop: "I can't go any further." They found an affordable motel and checked in. For several hours Stan and Ed took turns in the bathroom with diarrhea and vomiting. Stan ran a slight fever and both complained of a headache. Ed said he was chilly even though it was a very warm day. Both Ed and Stan complained of dizziness. Billy seemed well, but he was concerned about his buddies. Finally, he talked to the desk clerk, who recommended an urgent care clinic down the road. Billy took his pals to the clinic, where the doctor took their vital signs as well as a description of their symptoms. Indeed both had a slight fever. It seems that Stan and Ed both had egg salad sandwich and milk for lunch, but Billy had picked up a couple of packages of his favorite peanut butter crackers instead of the sandwich. He also had milk. All three picked up some grapes, but Billy had only a few since he was driving, while the other two had eaten quite a lot. All three enjoyed some homemade cookies the farmer's wife had baked that morning. They were oatmeal raisin cookies and were delicious.

Problem Analysis and Resolution

1. What do you think was the vector for this illness? How could this have been prevented by the farm store?

2. How long do you think these boys will be ill? What are some of the concerns the doctor might have?

3. What would be their best treatment option?

4. Would you suggest returning to Alabama or continuing on to Cancun? Why?

Case Study 9.2: Oh Those Tomatoes!

It is summer and lots of people are enjoying fresh tomato sandwiches. Many harvest toma-toes out of their backyard gardens, including Mattie Ray and Terry. They have a big garden every year. They have a small dairy farm along with a few yard chickens and manage to grow a large percentage of the food they consume using the traditional methods their par-ents and grandparents taught them. They try not to spend any money on soil amendments, preferring to raise their food crops organically. They think that the quality of the food they raise is far better than what can be found in the local supermarket. However, one day last August, Mattie Ray and Terry both began to feel "poorly." Their daughter happened by that day and was concerned. Both had lost weight and although the cows had been milked and minimal chores had been done, neither Terry nor Mattie Ray had done anything else. The house was a mess and both Terry and Mattie Ray complained of abdominal cramps, diar-rhea, fatigue, and anorexia. The garden was in full bloom with lots of fresh fruits and veg-etables but no one had been out to collect these goodies and they were rotting in place. The dung heap had not been shoveled out in several days and it was apparent that neither Terry nor Mattie Ray had been able to spread the manure on the fields or on the garden as was their practice. They liked the idea of using the fecal material as fertilizer so that they avoid using the inorganic fertilizer from the farm supply store. However, the last time they had spread the dung was several weeks ago. Since they did not have an indoor toilet, they also used the waste from their outhouse on their fields and garden. They were true recyclers!

Now Mattie Ray and Terry were sick. They hated to admit it, but they were bone tired and could not keep up the work on their farm. They needed help. Their daughter took them to the doctor's office and in turn the doctor sent them both to the hospital for tests and evaluations.

Problem Analysis and Resolution

1. What do you think the hospital did to investigate the problem with Terry and Mattie Ray? What would you do if you were in charge of the situation?

2. What do you think is the problem with Mattie Ray and Terry?

3. What strategies would you suggest to treat these people and prevent a recurrence?

Case Study 9.3: Jesse and His Family Get Sick

Mary's young son Jesse has had a difficult first year. His first few months after birth were relatively stress free. He grew and gained weight normally. Unfortunately, over the last several weeks, all the members of Jesse's family have had an intestinal virus that included vomiting and diarrhea. Jesse also had diarrhea and vomiting. One night Jesse woke the entire family with sudden loud crying. When Mary went to check on him, his legs were drawn up against his chest and he clearly demonstrated significant abdominal pain. The pain eventually passed but came back in the morning. That morning, Mary noticed that Jesse's stool was bloody and appeared to have some mucus in it. Jesse appeared pale, sluggish, sweaty, and had a fever. Mary took Jesse to the emergency room where radiography showed a telescoped intestine. This is called *intussusception* of the colon.

Problem Analysis and Resolution

Using the information above, answer the following questions:

1. What caused Jesse's intestine to telescope?

2. Why was Jesse pale and sluggish? What clinical remedy could be used to stabilize Jesse?

3. What does the blood and mucus in Jesse's stool indicate?

4. What are the treatment alternatives for Jesse? What sort of diet is needed for Jesse to recover normally?

chapter 10

Stones and Bones

Bone Mineralization

The skeleton is a complex, metabolically active tissue that serves multiple physiological functions. However, its most important purpose is to maintain normal stature and locomotion by virtue of its hardness. This quality is conferred by a unique arrangement of a calcium/phosphorus-containing mineral called *hydroxyapatite* embedded in a protein matrix composed predominately of type 1 collagen (90+%). The matrix also contains a large number of noncollagenous proteins, some of which are unique to bone. Altogether, the mineral and protein components confer both hardness and flexibility, which minimizes brittleness.

The human skeleton matures during growth and development by a process called *modeling*, during which the enlarging skeleton is repetitively resorbed via osteoclastic activity, and then reformed on a larger template by osteoblastic action. Once growth is complete, these same two opposing processes continue to operate in a coupled manner, so that areas of bone that have undergone microdamage due to the repetitive strain incurred by activities of daily living (plus work-related and athletic activities) can be continually replaced by new healthy bone. This process, which predominates in the adult, is known as *remodeling*, and when the two opposing processes of resorption of defunct bone and reformation of healthy bone are qualitatively and quantitatively coupled, the skeleton retains its normal strength and hardness.

Bone Diseases

Osteoporosis and osteomalacia are two diseases of the skeletal system and are sometimes referred to as *metabolic bone disease*. These diseases are actually disturbances in the orderly cascade of skeletal modeling and remodeling. Bone mineralization follows reformation of the matrix and is an osteoblastic controlled function. Table 10.1 gives examples of the more common metabolic bone diseases.

The coupling of bone resorption, reformation, and mineralization is normally orchestrated and modulated by a large repertoire of hormones, growth factors, resorptive cytokines, and miscellaneous factors (Table 10.2) that determine ultimate bone mass and anatomy, and resistance to fracture during casual trauma. Nutritional status is the key to the normal interactions among these factors, and in the evaluation of individuals in whom skeletal integrity is a clinical issue. The consideration of dietary status is a primary step, since all other interactions will be adversely affected by uncorrected dietary deficiencies. Table 10.3 is a list of the macro- and micronutrients that have a role in skeletal modeling and remodeling. Obviously, calcium leads the list of nutrients, since it is the most abundant mineral in bone. The skeleton accounts for greater than 90% of body calcium content (Table 10.4). The gastrointestinal (GI) absorption of calcium is affected by a large number of factors such as transit time, mucosal competence, other nutrients, and calcium binding by phosphates, oxalate, and fiber. However, vitamin D is the dominant factor influencing

Table 10.1 Metabolic Bone Diseases

- Disturbances in orderly sequence of skeletal turnover: resorption-formation-mineralization
- Examples:

↓resorption:	osteopetrosis
↓formation:	osteogenesis imperfecta
↓mineralization:	osteomalacia
↑resorption:	skeletal hyperparathyroidism
↑resorption, ↑formation:	Paget's disease
↑resorption, ↓formation:	osteoporosis

calcium absorption since its active metabolite, 1,25-dihydroxy-vitamin D (cholecalciferol) stimulates production of a specific calcium-binding protein (calbindin) in mucosal cells. Calbindin is responsible in the enterocytes for the absorption of calcium. This is especially important for older persons in whom several age-related deficits in vitamin D metabolism and action are common. Since the average nondairy diet contains only 300–500 mg of calcium, the intentional use of calcium-rich foods or a calcium supplement daily is necessary to meet need. Calcium supplements containing vitamin D are preferred if the individual does not consume sufficient dairy foods and expose the skin to sufficient sunlight for vitamin D synthesis. The use of sunscreens blocks vitamin D synthesis, so a vitamin D supplement is essential. When significant hepatic and/or renal disease is present, it may be necessary to substitute vitamin D metabolites such as 25,hydroxy-vitamin D or 1,25-dihydroxy vitamin D for the natural vitamin to ensure that sufficient active vitamin D is available to stimulate the uptake of calcium through the intestinal mucosa.

Other macronutrients critical to the skeleton include phosphorus (phosphate), magnesium, protein, and lipids. The average American who is not a vegetarian consumes sufficient phosphorus-rich foods and beverages so that a phosphorus deficiency is rarely a problem. In fact, excess phosphorus should be avoided since it may increase bone resorption by stimulating excess parathyroid hormone (PTH) release. Calcium phosphate supplements as a calcium source are not desirable, not only because of a possible stimulatory effect on PTH, but also because the excess phosphate may excessively bind calcium in the GI tract. Excess phosphate may also combine with calcium internally and facilitate its removal from the circulation by deposition within soft tissues and on bone surfaces. The latter does not necessarily contribute to bone integrity

Table 10.2 Hormones That Affect Bone Formation and Remodeling

Parathyroid hormone, biphasic effect: low dose, ↑ trabecular and cortical bone formation; high dose ↑ cortical and trabecular bone resorption.

Vitamin D increases calcium uptake and mineralization.

Calcitonin inhibits bone resorption and stimulates bone formation.

Corticosteroids inhibit bone formation and secondarily stimulate bone resorption.

Gonadal steroids inhibit bone resorption and stimulate bone formation.

Thyroid hormones increase bone turnover.

Growth hormone stimulates bone formation and resorption.

Insulin stimulates bone formation.

Prolactin inhibits bone formation.

Table 10.3 Nutrients Important to Bone Health

Vitamin K	Vitamin E
Calcium	Vitamin D
Phosphorus	Vitamin C
Magnesium	Vitamin A

except in undermineralized bone (osteomalacia) in which a high phosphorus intake is often beneficial.

The need for adequate protein of high biological value to ensure adequate production of bone collagen and noncollagenous bone proteins is obvious. Patients with eating disorders and protein-calorie malnutrition uniformly have deficient skeletons. Several nutrients that are variable components of the human diet can have important influences on the skeleton, affecting either calcium metabolism or the skeleton directly. Excess fiber, caffeine, and acid-containing foods and beverages all have negative effects, whereas the isoflavones and related compounds present in various foods are "weak estrogens" and exert a positive effect. Alcohol is technically not a nutrient, but is so ubiquitous in the human diet as to be considered so. An excess intake has multiple adverse actions on bone modeling and remodeling.

Aside from vitamin D, four other vitamins have been shown to have an influence on the skeleton. Vitamin A in excess and its more powerful retinoic acid derivatives (used to treat acne, other dermatological conditions, and certain neoplasms) are powerful stimulators of the osteoclast and can cause bone loss and even hypercalcemia. Vitamin C, however, is an osteoblast promoter, and severe deficiency sufficient to cause borderline scurvy is accompanied by bone lesions. Vitamin E also increases experimental bone formation, but its clinical significance has not been established. Vitamin K, as a cofactor for gamma-hydroxylation, is responsible for the production of osteocalcin, a noncollagenous matrix protein. Although low vitamin K levels have been reported in some people with osteoporosis, an etiological connection, if any, is unproven. A large number of trace elements have either positive or negative effects on the skeleton, but the majority are of interest in experimental systems and have no proven benefits or dangers to patients.

Osteoporosis

In osteoporosis there may be sufficient bone mineral loss to place patients at immediate risk for fracture. In this instance, it may be desirable to treat the bone disease pharmacologically. During nutrition counseling for osteoporosis, nonpharmacological approaches

Table 10.4 Composition of the Skeleton

The skeleton is approximately 8% of the total body weight. On a dry weight basis	
35% is organic:	Type 1 collagen (90+%)
	Noncollagenous proteins: Glycosaminoglycans, proteoglycans, glycoproteins, osteocalcin, osteonectin, osteopontin, bone sialoprotein, alkaline phosphatase, etc. Growth factors and cytokines and a small amount of lipid
65% is inorganic:	Hydroxyapatite: $Ca_{10}(PO_4)_6(OH)_2$
	Magnesium, sodium, potassium carbonate containing salts
	Fluorine plus some "heavy metals" and some trace elements

can be used. These include calcium–vitamin D supplements, exercise, and nutrition assessment to ascertain adequacy of nutrient intake. Falls are a particularly serious cofactor in fractures and are mostly preventable. Adequate protein-calorie nutrition promotes muscular strength and agility and therefore helps prevent falls. Although these recommendations are intended for primary types of osteoporosis, they are also applicable, with modifications, in secondary forms of osteoporosis. As an example, calcium and vitamin D intakes should be carefully monitored by serum and urine calcium measurements in hyperparathyroidism and idiopathic excess urine calcium. If urine calcium rises unduly, a thiazide diuretic could be used to reduce urine calcium excretion. In corticosteroid-induced osteoporosis, if the prednisone equivalent dose is 5 mg per day or higher, the vitamin D intake should be drastically increased to the range of 5000–7000 IU per day. The nonpharmacological approaches described are equally applicable to patients with lesser degrees of bone loss, so-called osteopenia. Advanced states of osteopenia may also qualify for a modified drug program.

Osteomalacia

There are many causes of osteomalacia, and most relate to defects in the vitamin D cascade or an endorgan resistance to active vitamin metabolites either genetic or acquired. Uncomplicated nutritional deficiencies (of calcium and/or vitamin D) are rare but do occur in the financially and socially stressed, and in the institutionalized elderly. A combination of calcium supplementation and active vitamin D is probably the most sensible approach to treating osteomalacia.

Skeletal Problems Associated with Renal Disease

The synthesis of active vitamin D occurs in the renal tissue. Hence it is not surprising that skeletal problems can develop in patients in renal failure. This is called *renal osteodystrophy*. It represents a variable combination of secondary hyperparathyroidism, osteomalacia, osteoporosis, and osteosclerosis. Nutritional therapy is an important aspect of treatment, although pharmacological and/or surgical approaches may also be necessary in particularly advanced cases. The aim is to suppress the secondary hyperparathyroidism and correct undermineralization by using maximally tolerated doses of the active metabolite of vitamin D, calcitriol (1,25-dihydroxy-vitamin D), and calcium. Calcium carbonate is preferred to calcium citrate, although both have the ability to bind phosphorus in the GI tract and thereby reduce the hyperphosphatemia, a major factor in the genesis of the renal osteodystrophy.

Other Diseases of the Bone

Skeletal abnormalities also occur in primary hyperparathyroidism. Previously, calcium restriction was advocated to lessen the impact of the hypercalcemia characteristic of the condition. However, the availability of bone density measurements has revealed that this results in greater bone loss and worsens the skeletal complications. Presently, adequate calcium and vitamin D intakes are advocated, preferably as food sources with a minimal use of supplements. The condition is best treated by surgery, although new pharmacological agents, called *calciomimetic* agents, are currently under development.

Another disease that affects the skeleton is Paget's disease. Although in this disease both bone resorption and formation are increased, their quantitative relationship is variable, so that either positive calcium balance (with hypocalciuria) or negative calcium balance (with hypercalciuria) may be present at any given time during the prolonged course of the condition. In any case, the imbalance rarely disturbs the serum calcium level and does not cause serious bone loss. Therefore, normal calcium and vitamin D intakes are the best approach, especially since having Paget's disease does not protect against osteoporosis. Since the bisphosphonates currently in use can occasionally cause transient, mild hypocalcemia, some authorities recommend an increased calcium intake during bisphosphonate treatment. However, calcium should not be supplemented if there is a history of calcium-containing kidney stones. Another type of stone that can occur in Paget's disease is the uric acid stone, since some patients also have a concomitant gout.

Renal Stone Disease

Urinary calculi, or kidney stones, form when inorganic salts precipitate and grow in size. These stones may be as small as grains of sand or may grow in size to that of small marbles. They can block the renal pelvis and staunch the flow of urine from the kidney to the bladder or from the bladder to the urinary tract. There are four major types of kidney stones. Cystine stones often coalesce to form large stones of a homogeneous wax-like appearance. Calcium oxalate stones may have a snowflake form with spicules radiating from a central point. Large staghorn stones are calcium phosphate or calcium carbonate. Uric acid, ureate, and cystine stones often fail to give a visible shadow upon x-ray. Each type has its own set of conditions under which it grows. Nutritional manipulation can slow the growth of these stones. However, stone recovery may be necessary to relieve the pain associated with their presence.

Types of Stones

There are several different types of stones. The most common is a calcium oxalate/phosphate stone. This stone type accounts for 80% of renal stones, and approximately 50% of these are idiopathic in that there is no discernible metabolic defect associated with their formation. In most patients with these stones, urinary calcium and oxalate levels are normal. In a few patients, either urinary calcium or oxalate is increased; the former may or may not be associated with hypercalcemia. Oxaluria may be a primary genetic condition, due to excessive intake of foods that yield oxalate during digestion or metabolism, or secondary to the increased oxalate absorption present in inflammatory bowel disease and in some malabsorption syndromes. In the cases related to gastrointestinal disease, intestinal calcium becomes bound to unabsorbed fats instead of luminal oxalate, allowing the latter to be absorbed and then excreted, followed by precipitation with calcium in the urinary tract. Calcium stones are difficult to treat, in the sense of preventing or reducing their rate of recurrence, because of their great insolubility. Successful treatment of an underlying medical condition, if present, is the most effective maneuver and should be combined with dietary changes consisting of manipulating the calcium intake, limiting vitamins A and D and oxalate intakes, and maintaining maximal hydration compatible with cardiovascular competence. In oxaluria, an increased calcium intake may allow more oxalate complexation in the gastrointestinal tract and actually lessen calcium oxalate stone formation. In the case of idiopathic hypercalciuria, an extreme reduction in calcium intake will have an adverse effect on bone density and increase the predisposition to osteoporosis/osteopenia.

The second type of stone is an $MgNH_4PO_4$ stone. In urinary tract infections caused by urea splitting organisms, both urine NH_4 levels and pH rise, and the NH_4 can combine with urinary Mg and PO_4 to precipitate in the alkaline medium. Lowering substrate excretion by dietary restriction and lowering pH using drugs that target urine acid-base balance will retard precipitation, but so long as the infection persists, NH_4 generation will limit the effectiveness of this manipulation. There are some highly effective drugs to treat these infections. Unfortunately, sometimes these infections are difficult to totally eradicate. The stones that are formed under these conditions can be quite large and irregularly shaped.

The third type of stone is the one in which cystine is involved. These are the rarest of kidney stones since they occur only in an inborn genetic condition, cystinuria. Although organic in composition, they are radio-opaque due to the dense packing of the cystine molecules. In mild cases, urinary alkalinization is successful, but when the stone disease is more aggressive, alkalinization must be combined with agents that can chelate the excess cystine.

Last, there are stones found in patients with gout. This is a uric acid-rich stone. This is the only major radiolucent stone, and its presence may need specialized imaging procedures. Patients with manifest gouty arthritis are particularly susceptible because of a combination of uricosuria and an intrinsic defect in urinary NH_3 production from purine precursors. These precursors force the kidney to excrete metabolically derived acids as titratable acidity, a condition under which uric acid is insoluble and can precipitate. A subset of patients exist in whom the urinary defect in NH_3 production is not accompanied by other features of the gouty diathesis, and these patients are easily treated with alkali supplements alone. A simple technique to detect these patients and to monitor alkali treatment is to have the patient record urinary pH of each voided specimen by placing pH-sensitive strips in the urinary stream. In normal individuals, pH will vary from 5.0 or less to 6.5 or higher (the "alkaline tide"), but patients with the defect will show persistent values of 5.0 or less throughout the 24 hours. With successful alkalinization, pH should remain at 6.0 or higher. Excessive purine intake (avoidance of oysters, shellfish, and liver) should be curtailed, but not at the expense of causing protein deficiency. Conditions associated with high catabolic states, such as burns, extensive trauma, and certain neoplasms, especially with the use of antineoplastic agents, can cause acute and severe hyperuricosuria, which may not only cause stone formation, but also clog the renal tubules, causing a "gouty nephropathy." Treatment with drugs to alkalinize the urine and forced hydration is required to forestall this serious complication. Paget's disease patients may also form uric acid stones because of the frequent tendency to a comorbid gouty diathesis, and should also receive careful alkalinization if this is a problem.

Sometimes a patient can present with stones of mixed origin. These represent a challenge in terms of diagnosis and treatment. Since treatment for one component may be deleterious for another component, a full understanding of the qualitative and quantitative nature of the metabolic defects present should be sought before instituting cautious treatment.

In addition to stones in the kidney are stones that form in the bladder. These stones are not those that have migrated to the bladder from the kidney. They are generally not related to metabolic defects, but to stasis. Their composition is variable and often a mixture of components. They are treated by correcting disturbed anatomy rather than dietary therapy.

Case Study 10.1: Aunt Tillie Is Getting Shorter

Aunt Tillie is 94 years old. She is mentally alert and emotionally stable. She has a problem, however. As the years have passed she has become shorter. Her niece, Nancy, noticed that whereas she used to be able to look Aunt Tillie in the eye, now she has to look down in order to meet Aunt Tillie's gaze. Aunt Tillie seems to have gotten frail as well. Concerned, Nancy took Aunt Tillie for a checkup. A dual energy x-ray absortiometry (DEXA) scan showed that for her age, Aunt Tillie's bones were reasonably dense—no real evidence of osteoporosis.

Problem Analysis and Resolution

1. Why is Aunt Tillie getting shorter? Discuss your reasons and speculate on the cause(s).

2. Are there any nutritional options that will help?

3. What strategies would you suggest that will make Aunt Tillie's life more comfortable?

Case Study 10.2: Mike Writhes on the Floor

Mike is a vigorous man, age 40, who enjoys the outdoors. He has a small horse farm and regularly works his horses. He also is a part-time builder, performing small renovation jobs for his friends and neighbors. One day as he was drinking coffee with his neighbor, he suddenly bent over and cried out in pain. The pain was so intense he was soon on the floor writhing in agony. His neighbor called 911 and Mike was rushed to the hospital. Pain relief was accomplished with some very heavy doses of medication and the doctors set about trying to find out the source of his pain.

Initially, Mike's pain began with a dull, intermittent discomfort in his flank and in the lumbar region of his back. Then it intensified across his abdomen as he was drinking coffee with his friend. It ran down the middle of his abdomen to his genitalia and to the inner aspect of his thigh. He began to sweat profusely, felt nauseous, and was faint. He teetered on the edge of shock. He felt the urge to urinate but very little urine was passed. By this time he was in the hospital and, with medication, the pain receded. A sample of urine was obtained. It was tinged with blood and there was evidence of albuminuria. An x-ray of his pelvic region was done but the shadows were inconclusive.

Problem Analysis and Resolution

1. What is Mike's problem?

2. What do you think the doctors will suggest by way of managing this problem?

3. Suggest some strategies that will be helpful to forestall future attacks.

Case Study 10.3: Bertha Takes a Fall

Bertha is 75 years old. One day as she was walking to her kitchen she fell. She was able to summon help and was transported to the hospital. X-rays of her hip revealed a fracture. She had not tripped or slipped and was puzzled as to the reason for her fall. Bertha was not overweight and she had been fairly active for a woman of her age.

Problem Analysis and Resolution

1. What is wrong with Bertha?

2. Why did she fall? Do you think the hip might have fractured before or after the fall?

3. What therapy do you think she might need to fully recover?

chapter 11

Age and Nutrition

The Aging Process

From the single fertilized cell to maturity and then senescence, the human passes through several important stages. From conception to birth is one of these, followed by the growth of infanthood and childhood, followed by adolescence. Each of these stages is characterized by both an increase in cell number and a concerted and coordinated change in cell/tissue/organ characteristics and function. Longitudinal growth of the skeleton is the most obvious feature accompanied by the growth and maturation of the muscles, the internal organs, the reproductive system, and the central nervous system. Once humans have attained maturity they maintain that stage for many decades; after that they slowly begin to decline with respect to their overall health and wellbeing. This is called *senescence*. Some people begin the stage of senescence earlier than others. Some adults are vigorous into their eighth and ninth decade of life while others are already senescent in their sixth decade. There are tremendous individual differences that in part are attributable to genetics and in part due to lifestyle choices and environmental effects.

During senescence there is a decrease in number of some cell types and a decline in function. Physical activity as well as the consumption of a well-balanced diet adequate in all the needed nutrients ensures not only a coordinated growth pattern but also an optimal maintenance at maturity. Should one or more of the essential nutrients be inadequate, optimal physiological status at maturity will be compromised. The elderly are the fastest growing segment in our population today. Citizens of Western, technologically advanced nations are living longer than their ancestors. In the United States, the segment of the population over the age of 65 has grown rapidly. For example, between 1960 and 1990, the total U.S. population increased by 39%. The segment of that population over the age of 65 grew by 89%. The segment of the population over the age of 84 grew by 232%. The elderly population segment is rising rapidly and with it are the health concerns that have implications with respect to nutrition.

As people age, many aspects of their lives change. Upon retirement, their income may be reduced and their healthcare expenses may increase. Age-related changes in the musculoskeletal systems of the elderly will probably mean less mobility. Older sensory systems may be less acute. Diminished senses of balance, hearing, smell, sight, and the overall perception of self in society have an impact on health and wellbeing, as well as on aging individuals' ability to care for themselves. The development of senile dementia of the Alzheimer's type, with subsequent losses in both mental and physical function, occurs more frequently as the population ages. With the significant gain in average life expectancy, a parallel rise in these age-related failures in brain function has occurred.

However, some deteriorated mental function might not be strictly age related. It might be due to malnutrition. Older adults may show signs of inadequate protein, mineral, and vitamin nutriture that impact their mental function. Inadequate intakes of vitamin B_{12}, folacin, and protein have been identified. When these inadequacies are addressed and nutritional status improved, some of the so-called age-related impaired mental functions are reversed.

Some malnutrition can be attributed to the loss of ability to purchase the needed food—either for economic reasons or because elders may not be able to get to the grocery store to select the foods they need and want. Their diminished sensory faculties may mean that they can no longer drive and thus must depend on their families and communities for their food supply. They may also be unable to prepare the food or store it appropriately, due to their diminished sensory function. If dentition is poor, the choice of foods might be limited to those items that are easy to swallow with minimal mastication. The absence of dentures or the presence of poorly fitted dentures can be a major impediment to the consumption of the wide variety of foods needed to ensure good nutritional status.

How can these problems be identified and corrected? This is not an easy question to answer. Nutrition screening of people over the age of 65 can present some special problems and hurdles. For a variety of reasons, many elders may not be able to read. Thus acquiring information about their usual food intake may have this additional complication. Short-term memory loss may cause some elderly people to be unable to recall the food they consumed yesterday or the day before. If elders are blind or have failing vision, they may not be able to complete a diet-recall form or compile a food-intake diary. Early indications of malnutrition are usually observed where the elders are receiving good medical care, while these indicators are ignored when little or no care is provided. Thus anemia due to mineral or vitamin deficiency or other nutrition-related maladies might be diagnosed readily in a good medical care setting and might be corrected, while these symptoms might be ignored when little or no care is provided. Osteoporosis, arthritis, and other degenerative diseases that have a nutrition component likewise could be identified and effectively treated along with other age-related problems when the elderly person is receiving regular medical care.

Good geriatric care also includes the recognition that some of the medications used in managing such chronic diseases as hypertension or diabetes mellitus may interact with certain nutrients, thus placing the patient at risk for malnutrition. Thiazide diuretics, for example, are widely prescribed for the management of hypertension. They are excellent medications for this purpose, but they increase the loss of potassium and frequently the elderly need to supplement their diets with potassium-rich foods (citrus fruits, bananas, etc.) or take a potassium supplement. The elderly may develop chemical imbalances in the brain that affect their emotional state. It is not unusual for physicians to prescribe antidepressants, and some of these drugs affect appetite as well as metabolism. Those drugs that are anticholinergics can have the side effects of dry mouth, altered taste perception, nausea, vomiting, constipation, and reduced appetite. All of these side effects can affect nutritional status because of their influence on food consumption. Similarly, nutritional status can be affected by the use of antacids and laxatives. Some of the elderly believe that a daily large bowel movement is essential. Despite day-to-day variation in the kinds and amounts of foods consumed, there is this belief that a daily movement is a feature of good health. Thus many elderly are chronic laxative users. This use may disturb gastrointestinal function and promote diarrhea as well as the possibility of an electrolyte imbalance. In turn, this will reduce gut passage time and thus absorptive cell exposure time for nutrients. Again, this can result in impaired nutritional status.

Diseases of the joints and connective tissue are frequently managed with the use of anti-inflammatories. Both steroids and nonsteroidal anti-inflammatory drugs are used to reduce the inflammation and associated pain. Aspirin and indomethacin are among the nonsteroidal, over-the-counter medications frequently used. If used daily in large doses, both can result in iron-deficiency anemia. High aspirin intake can deplete the hepatic iron stores. The elderly can have bruises and small "bleeds" that result in blood loss and anemia. A number of other drugs can influence nutritional status. However, many drugs have not been studied at all with respect to their effect on nutritional status, especially in the elderly. Nonetheless, interest in drug–nutrient interactions is building as we learn more about the gradual losses in body function that characterize aging.

Age-Related Changes in Metabolism

Aging in itself has effects on the pathways of intermediary metabolism as well as on the endocrine system. These effects are listed in Table 11.1. Insulin resistance may be a feature of aging. With age the pancreas becomes less responsive to signals for insulin release and the target tissues become less responsive to its action. In part this may be due to age-related increased plasma membrane phospholipid saturation, but it is also due to age-related increase in fat cell size. As fat cells accumulate stored fat they become less responsive to the action of insulin in promoting glucose uptake and use. Muscle cells likewise may have age-related changes in membrane fluidity that impair their response to insulin. With age there is a decrease in muscle activity as people become more sedentary. Active or working muscle is not as dependent on insulin for glucose use as are nonworking muscles.

Altogether this decrease in muscle activity plus the increase in fat cell size has a negative effect on the insulin–glucose relationship. Glucose levels rise and the β cells of the pancreatic islets of Langerhans increase their output of insulin to meet the glucose challenge. However, this excess output does little good in reducing the blood glucose in the aging, overly fat, inactive individual and it is not uncommon to have type 2 diabetes develop as a consequence. Age-related impaired glucose tolerance can be mitigated by food restriction and increased activity, which reverses the above physiological state. Because insulin is one of the main regulators of intermediary metabolism and because its action is counterbalanced by the glucocorticoids, the catecholamines, the thyroid hormones, glucagon, and several other hormones, it should be no surprise that age changes in these hormones occur as well. Again, some of these changes can be attributed to age changes in membrane lipids, but some can be attributed to changes in hormone production and in the synthesis and activity of the receptors that mediate their action. Table 11.2 lists some hormones affected by age. The blood levels of most of these hormones decrease in the aging human. A few pass through a phase where they are elevated above normal, then fall below normal as aging continues. All of these hormones serve to regulate the metabolism of carbohydrate, lipid, and protein. In humans, age has effects on voluntary food intake. In a number of instances the age-related decline in activity of a pathway or reaction is less in the lean person than in the person with excess fat stores. The lean person probably self-restricts his/her food intake so as to remain lean. Perhaps this food restriction is innate. That is, the individual is unaware that the food intake is such that body fat stores are minimized. There may be internal signals that actively promote food restriction and suppress excess consumption.

Table 11.1 Age Effects on Metabolic Pathways

Glucose use	decrease
Glycogen synthesis	no change
Glycogen use	no change
Glucose synthesis	increase
Fat synthesis	increase
Fat mobilization	decrease
Protein synthesis	decrease

Table 11.2 Hormone Changes with Age

Hormone	Effects with Age
Thyroxine (T$_4$)	↓
Triiodothyronine (T$_3$)	↓
Thyroid binding globulin	No change or ↑
Thyroid stimulating hormone (TSH)	↓
Insulin	↑ followed by ↓
ACTH	↓
Epinephrine	↓
Glucagon	↓
Growth hormone	↓
Estrogen	↓
Testosterone	↓
Cortisol (Glucocorticoids)	↓
Pancreatic polypeptide	↓

↑ *increase;* ↓ *decrease*

This inhibition of aging by a reduction in food intake probably has to do with the decreased fat stores that are the result of such a feeding pattern. A decrease in fat store reduces the supply of fatty acid precursors for free radical production and in turn this may lead to a reduction in free radical damage to vital cellular components. Some have suggested that as free radical increases there are increases in damage to genetic material as well as protein damage with resultant loss of function. In addition, a reduced fat store has effects on peripheral cell responsivity to insulin vis-à-vis glucose use, and, of course, in the absence of hyperinsulinemia, there is a decreased release of the anti-insulin hormones. These changes all affect glucose homeostasis.

As aging proceeds there can be a rise in blood lipids coupled with a decrease in adipose tissue lipoprotein lipase. With age, adipocytes have a less competent lipid uptake system due to this decline in lipase activity. In normal-aging animals the rates of cholesterol synthesis do not change; however, the uptake of this cholesterol as well as its oxidation and excretion declines. This has the result of an age-related increase in serum cholesterol levels. Genetics plays an important role in these age-related changes in serum lipids. Some genotypes are characterized by a sharper decline with age in lipid uptake processes than other genotypes. Some may only have a decline in cholesterol uptake or triacylglyceride uptake, while others will have a decline in the uptake of both. Age-related declines in thyroid hormone production, thyroxine conversion to triiodothyronine, glucocorticoid release, and the insulin:glucagon ratio will have effects on fatty acid mobilization and oxidation, and the results of this decline in hormone-stimulated lipolysis are observed as an age-related expansion of the fat stores. In the young animal there is considerable protein synthesis and with age there is a decline in this synthetic activity. With an age-related decline in protein synthesis there is an increased need to rid the body of amino groups as the surplus amino acids are deaminated for use in gluconeogenesis and lipogenesis. This means that if the protein intake is not reduced to accommodate the decreased need for protein, there will be an increase in the activity of the urea cycle. Whether all of these effects on metabolism and hormonal balance are truly age related or due to other factors (disease, drugs, loneliness, etc.) is difficult to assess. Human studies are limited in the variables that can be manipulated in order to study the effects of aging on these measurements.

Case Study 11.1: Grandma Is Tired

Grandma is 70 years old. Lately she has been complaining of feeling tired. Whereas she used to enjoy working outside in her garden, she no longer does so and her garden is full of weeds. Her beautiful flowers are disappearing as the weeds take over. Grandma no longer wants to go shopping. She goes to the store for her groceries but minimizes the number of items she buys. She says she is too tired to carry all those groceries home, but her grandson, Allan, thinks she may not be able to afford both food and the medications she needs to manage her hypertension. Grandma also complains of joint stiffness and, reluctantly, she admits to using large amounts of aspirin to control her joint pain. Allan decides that Grandma should go to her doctor for evaluation. The doctor orders x-rays to determine the cause of the joint pain and also a blood workup to determine what other factors might cause her tiredness.

Problem Analysis and Resolution

1. What do you think the x-rays will show?

2. What do you think the doctor ordered in the way of blood tests and what do you think the results will be?

3. What do you suspect may be the cause of the tiredness? What systems are involved in this problem and how have they failed?

4. Discuss Grandma's situation and the strategies you would employ if she were your Grandma.

Case Study 11.2: Lydia Has Palpitations

Lydia is a retired nurse. She is 63 years old. As a child she had rheumatic fever. At the age of 34 she had a mitral valve replaced. She is 10% over her ideal body weight. She used to be quite active when she was working, but she has slowed down a lot with retirement. She has noticed bouts of dizziness and sometimes she thought she was close to fainting. Other times her heart seemed to race. She thought that maybe she needed to see a cardiologist and so she set up an appointment for a cardiac evaluation. Her examination included x-rays, EKG, blood pressure measurement, and a full cardiac workup. The results showed a mild pulmonary congestion, an enlarged left atrium and ventricle. Cardiac output was 3.0 L/min, blood pressure was 101/57, left atrial pressure was 17 mm Hg, and the right ventricular pressure was 44/8 mm Hg. The EKG indicated an atrial arrhythmia and there appeared to be some valvular regurgitation when the cardiologist listened to her heart sounds.

Problem Analysis and Resolution

1. Based on the information provided what do you think is going on? Do you think there is any relationship between the present condition and the history of rheumatic fever? If so, explain the relationship. If not, why not?

2. Define the terms *arrhythmia, tachycardia,* and *fibrillation*. What can explain the arrhythmia? The tachycardia? What is the significance of the fibrillation?

3. What is the outlook for this 63-year-old woman?

4. What would you suggest as a strategy for improving her health as she ages?

5. Do you think this problem has anything to do with her blood lipids or her diet?

chapter 12

Getting from Here to There—Muscle

One of the chief characteristics of the animal kingdom is its ability to move from place to place. While plants are stationary, animals move about. This characteristic is attributable to the bones and muscles working together under the control of the central nervous system. Chapter 10 addressed the skeletal system, so, except for the fact that the muscles are attached to the bones, that system will not be addressed in this chapter.

Muscle accounts for ~40% of the body weight in the adult human. It also can account for a significant portion of the daily energy need. Active working skeletal muscle uses glucose as its metabolic fuel and, in this condition, does not require insulin bound to its membrane receptor to facilitate glucose use. Resting muscle does require insulin for its glucose use. Muscle can also use fatty acids as an energy source but this use is very limited. Muscle mass can be increased through regular use, and further increases can be achieved by training of the muscles, as in athletic training for competitive sports. Training results in an increase in muscle oxygen use, an increase in energetic efficiency, a decrease in insulin-dependent glucose use, a loss in extra fat reserves, and as already mentioned, an increase in muscle mass. People who incorporate physical activity in their daily lives reap some of these same benefits. They are better able to control their appetite, better able to maintain a normal body weight, and better able to avoid stress, as well as delay the onset of degenerative diseases such as diabetes and cardiovascular disease. It should come as no surprise, therefore, that people should incorporate physical activity into their daily lives as a way of increasing energy expenditure and keeping glucose levels within the normal range.

Types of Muscle and Their Function

The skeletal muscle is essentially a pulling system, not a pushing one. That is, the muscles contract but do not expand. They can relax after contraction. Anatomically, for every skeletal muscle contraction there must also be an opposing skeletal muscle that will contract so that the initial muscle can relax and recover. Thus there are pairs of muscle fibers in every location in the skeletal system that alternate in action.

Muscle either has many mitochondria or fewer mitochondria. If the muscle has many mitochondria, it is a red muscle, whereas if there are fewer mitochondria, it is a white muscle. Some of the major skeletal muscle groups in the body are mixtures of red and white muscle. Individual muscle cells are called *myocytes*.

When muscle mass is increased as through use, both red and white skeletal muscles are increased in size. All of the skeletal muscles are striated. That is, one can see bands within the muscle when that muscle is examined microscopically. Striated muscle consists of many multinucleated fiber cells surrounded by an electrically excitable membrane, the sarcolemma. The bundles of fibers are embedded in a fluid called the sarcoplasm. The sarcoplasm contains a variety of electrolytes, glycogen, the enzymes of intermediary metabolism, and the high-energy compounds creatine phosphate and ATP. The muscle unit is called a *sarcomere*. Both skeletal muscle and the heart muscle are striated muscles.

Muscles that are associated with the internal organs are primarily white muscle; they are the smooth nonstriated muscles associated with organs such as the gastrointestinal tract, kidneys, bladder, gallbladder, and the lungs. Cardiac muscle, in contrast to the skeletal muscle groups and the white, smooth muscles, is unique. It resembles skeletal muscle in that it has many mitochondria and is striated, but it differs from skeletal muscle in that it has an intrinsic rhythmicity. The individual cardiac myocytes communicate with each other because of their syncytial nature. A syncytium is a multinucleated protoplasmic mass formed by the secondary union of individual cells. The muscle fibers appear to be interconnected and function as though they are. The cardiac muscle contracts in response to a signal generated by the atrial-ventricle (A-V) node located on the right side of the heart; first the upper chambers (the atria) contract and send blood to the lower chambers (the ventricles), and then the ventricles contract. The muscle is highly dependent on the calcium ion for contraction. It is also dependent on adequate supplies of high-energy compounds.

Both the skeletal muscle and the cardiac muscle are characterized by thick and thin filaments. The thick filaments contain the protein myosin, and the thin ones contain the proteins, actin, tropomyosin, and troponin. Under the electron microscope muscle fibers appear to have many bands. These bands differ in appearance based on whether they are thick or thin filaments. They have been designated as the A band and the I band. Thick filaments are confined to the A band and are arranged hexagonally if examined in a cross-section of the muscle. The filaments are about 16 nm in diameter. The other filament, the thin one, extends into the A band, but not into the H region of the A band. The thin filaments are arranged around the thick ones and usually there are three thick filaments to every thin one in the center of the muscle fiber, whereas each thick filament is surrounded by six thin filaments on the outside of the fiber. These thick and thin filaments interact through the formation of bridges that emerge every 14 nm along the thick filament. When the muscle is stimulated to contract, the bridges slide across the thick filament and the muscle shortens. As the muscle relaxes, the bridges slide back to their original positions. This is a very simplistic explanation of muscle contraction. Layered on top of this explanation is the role of the calcium ion and energy from creatine phosphate and ATP.

Calcium leaves its storage place on the sarcoplasmic reticulum and travels to the mitochondria whereupon it stimulates the release of ATP. The ATP provides energy to reform the creatine phosphate that was used to initiate the contraction of the muscle. Energy is needed as the filaments slide toward each other and form bridges. When the muscle relaxes, the high-energy compounds used must be resynthesized and the calcium ion sent back to the sarcoplasmic reticulum. If the calcium is not sent back, rigor (permanent contracture) develops. This is what happens in rigor mortis. Muscle cramps are another form of this contracture. These can occur when the muscle lacks sufficient oxygen for its mitochondria, which in turn use the oxygen to make water and ATP. Some of this cramping might also be due to a relative shortage of magnesium. Magnesium is an important player in the movement of the calcium ion both to its transport into the cell and its movement from the sarcoplasmic reticulum to the muscle mitochondrial compartment and return. Magnesium deficiency in pigs has been shown to result in muscle rigor. This has not been shown in humans.

Muscle is the major transducer of the body. It converts the chemical energy of creatine phosphate and ATP into mechanical energy. As described above, it requires the calcium ion and a constant energy supply (from glucose oxidation) to form and reform creatine phosphate and ATP. It also must be regulated; that is, it cannot work indefinitely.

Its speed, duration, and force must be controlled such that with every contraction there is a relaxation. This control is exerted by the neural system that dictates speed, duration, and force. Control is also exerted by the fuel supply; if there is insufficient fuel the muscle will tire. Muscle uses not only the glucose from the circulation but also the glucose from the small glycogen store present in the muscle. Should the muscle be unable to use its glycogen store, the individual will be unable to exercise. This inability to exercise is the key symptom of people with glycogen storage disease. These people synthesize glycogen but are unable to break it down. There are several mutations that phenotype as glycogen storage disease.

How Nutrition Affects Muscle Function

Despite the firm belief by athletic trainers and exercise coaches, a diet with an excess of protein beyond that needed by the body to sustain its protein metabolism has no effect on muscle mass or strength. Athletic performance is not affected by excess protein intake. If the athlete consumes an adequate diet containing all the essential nutrients in the amounts determined to be satisfactory for that athlete, then any additional amount will simply be degraded and excreted. Protein supplements usually are a waste of money if the diet of the athlete already contains the needed amounts of protein. The daily recommended intake for protein by various age groups can be found at the National Academy of Sciences Web site: www.nap.edu.

Increased use of the skeletal muscle does increase the energy requirement. You can calculate your energy requirement by first calculating your basal energy need (your BMR) using one of several formulas. The most common is the Harris Benedict formula. There are different ones for men and women:

$$BMR = 66.4730 + 13.751W + 5.0033L - 6.750A \text{ (men)}$$

$$BMR = 655.0955 + 9.563W + 1.8496L - 4.6756A \text{ (women)}$$

where W = weight in kg; L = height in cm; A = age in years.

Although excess protein intake and excess intake of other essential nutrients are generally considered ineffective with respect to muscle function, the opposite is not true when it comes to undernutrition or malnutrition. Both insufficient nutrition and starvation result in a loss of muscle mass and subsequent losses in endurance and the ability to do work. Deficient intake of the B vitamins results in anemia and also results in a decreased supply of those nutrients that serve as coenzymes in muscle metabolism. Inadequately nourished individuals therefore are less able to function efficiently with respect to movement and work. The muscles will not receive enough oxygen because of the anemia, nor will they have adequate supplies of energy, coenzymes, and cofactors (essential minerals) needed for muscle metabolism. If the diet is inadequate in protein, there will be insufficient supplies of amino acids available for the replenishment of muscle cells as they need replacement. Although muscle cells have a much longer half-life than do the red blood cells, they do need replenishment. Cells apoptose (natural cell death) and are replaced. The protein in the myocytes turns over and must be resynthesized using amino acids from the body pool. Heavy work increases the need to resynthesize the muscle protein. Malnourished individuals are less likely to have these needed amino acids for muscle cell repair and replacement.

Muscle Problems

There are a number of abnormalities in muscle metabolism that have been noted. One is a group of diseases called *muscular dystrophy*. In this condition the muscle fails to grow and regenerate normally. Muscle weakness is the prominent feature together with an early death. There are a number of genetic mutations that account for this disease. Most of these are carried on the X chromosome, and so most of the victims are male. There is a less severe form that is an autosomal mutation rather than a sex-linked mutation. It is quite rare and can occur in both males and females. The clinical features of these diseases are, in addition to muscle weakness and failure to thrive, an elevated creatine kinase, muscle necrosis (muscle death), and some variation in the size of the remaining muscle fibers. Studies of the DNA of patients with these disorders have revealed mutations in several places. For the patients with Duchenne muscular dystrophy there is a deletion in the code for dystrophin. This is a protein that is important for muscle protein resynthesis and cell renewal. It is also important in the contraction/relaxation function of the muscle. At this time it is not possible to correct these genetic problems. Perhaps in the future there will be technologies available for effective treatment.

Another disease of the muscle is a condition known as *malignant hyperthermia*. Under normal conditions, this is not a life-affecting disease. Yet, should a person having this problem have halothane anesthesia, it could result in death. The condition is associated with an abnormal accumulation of the calcium ion in the cytoplasm of muscle cells. There is a mutation in the gene for the calcium channel in the sarcoplasmic reticulum. Calcium ion movement from the sarcoplasmic reticulum to the mitochondria is an important aspect in mitochondrial metabolism. It is an essential feature for the regeneration of ATP. Should the regeneration of ATP be inhibited, excess heat will be released because the energy of the high-energy bond of the ATP has not been captured. Hence, the name for this condition is *malignant hyperthermia*. This causes muscle rigor and if not promptly recognized and treated, will cause death. Not only are humans affected by this disorder, but it has also been recognized in swine. In these animals it can cause significant financial loss to the farmer because it results in a condition known as *soft pork*. In pigs the response is elicited by stress. For example, if the pigs are subjected to high environmental temperature and if they have this genetic disorder, they will develop soft muscle tissue.

Although heart disease is a disease usually associated with loss in elasticity of the vascular system due to plaque formation, heart disease involves both the vascular system and the cardiac muscle. When the blood supply is cut off via an occlusion of the blood vessels that supply it, an area of the heart muscle dies. It can no longer respond to the electrical signal sent from the AV node that signals contracture. This is called a myocardial infarction because there is an interruption in this electrical wave that usually spreads across the muscle. Depending on the size of the infarction, the efficiency of the pumping action of the heart is mildly, moderately, or severely impaired. In the general population heart failure may be the end stage of cardiovascular disease preceded by heart attack(s) that have cut off the blood supply to various portions of the heart. Heart disease is the leading cause of death in Western nations.

Heart failure is a very common medical condition that arises from a variety of causes. In some instances the heart failure is due to genetically induced cardiomyopathies. Mutations in the genes for the β-myosin heavy chain have been identified as being associated with familial hypertrophic cardiomyopathy. Cardiomyopathy has also been shown to be a response to some cancer drugs as well as to mutations in some of the mitochondrial genes.

Learning Activity 12.1: Your Basal Energy Need

Calculate your basal energy need using the Harris Benedict formula. The results are given as kcals/kg/hour. Multiply this number by 24 to have an estimate of your daily basal energy need per kilogram. Now multiply by your weight in kilograms.

1. Convert your weight to kilograms (divide your weight in pounds by 2.2).

2. Convert your height in inches to centimeters (multiply inches by 25.4).

3. What is your daily basal energy need?

Learning Activity 12.2: Activity Cost

Keep a 3-day diary of all of your activities, including sleep. Using the figures from Table 12.1 estimate the energy cost of these activities. The energy associated with sleep is 90% of the basal energy that you estimated in Learning Activity 12.1. Add all of the energy costs (except that of sleep) of your activities. Divide by 3 since you are to keep a 3-day record. That will be the average energy cost of your activities. To get the total for your energy need, add the cost of the activity energy to the basal energy and then add the energy cost of sleep. This will give you an estimate of your energy expenditure for a 24-hour period.

Now then, you acquired an estimate of your energy consumption earlier in the book. How close are your two estimates?

Do you need to adjust one or the other to lose or gain weight? How or what would you do?

Table 12.1 Energy Cost of Activities, Exclusive of Basal
Metabolism and the Influence of Food

Activity	kcal/kg/h	(kJ/kg/h)
Bedmaking	3.0	12.6
Bicycling (century .run)	7.6	31.9
Bicycling (moderate .speed)	2.5	10.5
Boxing	11.4	47.9
Carpentry (heavy)	2.3	9.7
Cello playing	1.3	5.5
Cleaning windows	2.6	10.9
Crocheting	0.4	1.7
Dancing, moderately active	3.8	16
Dancing, rhumba	5.0	21
Dancing, waltz	3.0	12.6
Dishwashing	1.0	4.2
Dressing and undressing	0.7	2.9
Driving car	0.9	3.8
Eating	0.4	1.7
Exercise, very light	0.9	3.8
Exercise, light	1.4	5.6
Exercise, moderate	3.1	13
Exercise, severe	5.4	22.7
Exercise, very severe	7.6	31.9
Fencing	7.3	30.7
Football	6.8	28.6
Gardening, weeding	3.9	16.4
Golf	1.5	6.3
Horseback riding, walk	1.4	5.9
Horseback riding, trot	4.3	18.0
Horseback riding, gallop	6.7	28.0
Ironing (5-lb. iron)	1.0	4.2

Table 12.1 Energy Cost of Activities, Exclusive of Basal
Metabolism and the Influence of Food (Continued)

Activity	kcal/kg/h	(kJ)
Knitting, sweater	0.7	2.9
Laboratory work	2.1	8.8
Laundry, light	1.3	5.4
Lying still, awake	0.1	0.4
Office work, standing	0.6	2.5
Organ playing (1/3 handwork)	1.5	6.3
Painting furniture	1.5	6.3
Paring potatoes	0.6	2.5
Piano playing (Mendelssohn's *Song Without Words*)	0.8	3.3
Piano playing (Beethoven's *Appassionata*)	1.4	5.9
Piano playing (Liszt's *Tarantella*)	2.0	8.4
Playing cards	0.5	2.1
Playing pingpong	4.4	18.4
Reading aloud	0.4	1.7
Rowing	9.8	41.0
Rowing in race	16.0	66.9
Running	7.0	29.3
Sawing wood	5.7	23.8
Sewing, hand	0.4	1.7
Sewing, foot-driven machine	0.6	2.5
Sewing, electric machine	0.4	1.7
Singing in loud voice	0.8	3.3
Sitting quietly	0.4	1.7
Skating	3.5	14.6
Skiing (moderate speed)	10.3	43.1
Standing at attention	0.6	2.5
Standing relaxed	0.5	2.1
Sweeping with broom, bare floor	1.4	5.9
Sweeping with carpet sweeper	1.6	6.7
Sweeping with vacuum sweeper	2.7	11.3
Swimming (2 mi/h)	7.9	33.1
Tailoring	0.9	3.8
Tennis	5.0	20.9
Typing, rapidly	1.0	4.2
Typing, electric typewriter	0.5	2.1
Violin playing	0.6	2.5
Walking (3 mi/h)	2.0	8.4
Walking rapidly (4 mi/h)	3.4	14.2
Walking at high speed (5.3 mi/h)	8.3	34.7
Washing floors	1.2	5.0
Writing	0.4	1.7

Learning Activity 12.3: Exploring Performance-Enhancing Products

Choose a performance-enhancing food product. Examine its nutrient content. Using the information you have gathered about your personal nutrient needs and energy expenditure, evaluate whether such a product would be a benefit to you.

Case Study 12.1: Jason Is a Cyclist

Jason used to weigh 250 pounds but he was only 5′9″ tall. Needless to say, he was carrying around a lot of extra weight. At the age of 18 he decided that he had carried around this weight for far too long and decided he was going to slim down. First he carefully reduced his food intake and began to walk. Gradually he increased his walking such that he was walking about 2 miles a day. He then increased the speed of his walking so that instead of taking an hour it took about 30 minutes. As he was starting college in the fall he thought that even this was taking too much time so he began to cycle. Oh, he really enjoyed the cycling! Of course, with this activity and his careful dieting he achieved his goal of losing 75 pounds. Now that cycling was a part of his life he realized he could cycle competitively. He would cycle to all his classes on campus, and whenever he had a spare hour or two he would train to increase his speed and agility. Now he was a lean cycling machine weighing 175 pounds and he reveled in his new look. As an additional incentive, he began to compete professionally and won prize money. This helped him with his college expenses and gave him a way to release all the tension and stress student life accorded. Much to his delight, he could feast on some of the forbidden foods he had had to give up when he first began to change his dieting and physical activity program.

Problem Analysis and Resolution

1. Describe the metabolic changes Jason went through as he went from 250 pounds to 175 pounds.

2. What was his muscle fuel choice initially and what is it now?

3. Has his muscle mass changed?

4. What is his energy need now and how has this changed with his change in lifestyle?

Case Study 12.2: *Jackson Aspires to Play Professional Football*

All through high school Jackson played football. His coach urged him to eat lots of energy-rich foods so that he would gain weight. His coach thought that weight would equal athletic ability and assigned Jackson to a spot on the team that would use this weight against the opponents' running backs. Jackson was taught to tackle his opponents and use his weight to keep them down. Jackson did not do a lot of running himself but relied on others to bring the opponents to him. Jackson was pretty good and soon colleges and universities began soliciting his application to their institution so he could play football for them. Jackson continued to eat to excess and soon he weighed 285 pounds and stood 6′ tall. Although some tackles were taller, none outweighed him.

As a junior in college, he began to feel tired after a workout. He no longer had the energy to run around and indulge in horseplay with the other guys. He would sit back and watch his teammates have a good time but he simply did not have the energy to indulge. Here he was at the age of 20 feeling like he was 70 years old! One day during a training session he told the coach and other trainers that he felt too tired to work out. They were concerned and sent him to the team doctor for a thorough physical.

Problem Analysis and Resolution

1. What do you think the doctor found? How do you think the physician would approach the problem?

2. If you were the physician what would you recommend?

3. What do you think are Jackson's chances of playing professional football given his current physical condition?

4. What would you think his future holds for him given his present state of health?

Case Study 12.3: Tonya Has a Heart Attack

Tonya is 68 years old. She is not overweight but she does have type 2 diabetes mellitus, which she controls with exercise and diet. She is physically active, keeping her home and garden in wonderful condition. One day as she was entering the grocery store she felt this terrible burning sensation up the middle of her chest and she collapsed. The ambulance was called and she went to the emergency room. Tonya had had a heart attack. When an EKG was performed there was an infarction found, and clearly she was in trouble. A calcium blocker was administered, as was some nitroglycerin. She was heavily sedated and placed on bed rest.

Problem Analysis and Resolution

1. What did the calcium blocker do? Why was it helpful?

2. What did the nitroglycerine do? Why was it helpful?

3. What happened to the heart muscle when this event occurred? Will the muscle recover? If so, what will happen to it and how will the recovery develop?

Case Study 12.4: Edward Enlists in the Army

Edward is so enthusiastic about joining the Army. He enlisted as soon as he was of age. He was accepted after a routine physical. He was neither overweight nor underweight. He was of average body build and height. When he got to boot camp after the preliminary induction procedures, the physical training began. Edward soon realized that he had no endurance at all. He certainly did not want to be viewed as a slacker, but he simply could not run or even walk long distances. His drill sergeant berated him unmercifully. One day as the troop was hiking, Edward collapsed. He was taken by the medics to the base hospital. The physicians there could not find anything wrong except that his blood glucose was very low. They then sent him to a larger more sophisticated army hospital where it was discovered that he had one of the milder forms of glycogen storage disease where the muscle was affected but not the liver. He could not mobilize his muscle glycogen store.

Problem Analysis and Resolution

1. Describe the muscle metabolic pattern in Edward that was different from normal.

2. Why did this problem appear at this time and not prior to army training?

3. What strategy could Edward use to avoid another exhaustion episode?

Glossary

Acetone	A three-carbon ketone found in small amounts in many tissues including blood. Large amounts are not normal; uncontrolled diabetes mellitus has elevated blood and urine ketones as an important symptom.
Acetylcholine	A neurotransmitter; it initiates changes in ion permeability at the neuromuscular junction.
Acidic amino acids	Amino acids having two carboxyl groups.
Acidosis	When the pH of the body drops below its normal pH of 7.4.
ACTH	Adrenocorticotropin. A hormone released by the pituitary that stimulates the release of adrenal hormones, the glucocorticoids (cortisol, cortisone, and corticosterone), and the mineralcorticoid, aldosterone.
Active immunity	Production of antibodies by an individual exposed to an antigen.
Active site (of a hormone, enzyme, or reactant)	The location within a reactive molecule where reaction occurs.
ADH (antidiuretic hormone or vasopressin)	Hormone that stimulates water reabsorption by the kidney.
Adipocytes	Fat cells.
Aldosterone	A steroid hormone produced by the adrenal cortex. This hormone stimulates the reabsorption of sodium by the kidney.
Alkalosis	When the body pH rises above pH 7.4.
Allergens	Substances that elicit an immunological response.
Alopecia	Loss of hair.
Alveoli	Cells in the lungs responsible for O_2/CO_2 exchange.
Amenorrhea	Cessation of menses.
Amino acids	Small organic compounds containing an amino group ($-NH_3$) and a carboxy group ($-COOH$).
Anabolic reactions	Reactions where large molecules are made from small ones; the process is called *anabolism*.
Androgens	Male sex hormones.
Anemia	Below-normal amounts of hemoglobin and/or red blood cells.

Aneurism   A bulge in the vascular tree.

Angina pectoris   Chest pain due to a lack of oxygen supplied to the heart muscle.

Anion   An electrolyte with a negative charge.

Anosmia   Loss of the sense of smell.

Anoxia   Lack of oxygen in blood or tissues.

Antibiotics   Drugs that inhibit or kill pathogens.

Antibodies   Soluble proteins (immunoglobulins) that have specific recognition sequences for specific antigens.

Anticoagulants   Compounds that interfere with blood clotting.

Antigen-presenting cell (APC)   Any cell that functions to present antigens to T-cells.

Antigens   Substances that are recognized as "foreign" by the body and that elicit the production of antibodies.

Antiport   An exit route for an ion from a cell or cell compartment.

Anus   Opening at the posterior end of the rectum.

Aphagia   Not eating.

Apoptosis   Programmed cell death; a natural part of the cell cycle.

Arrhythmia   Abnormal (irregular) heart rhythms.

Aseptic   Sterile; absence of pathogens.

Atherosclerosis, arteriosclerosis   A progressive degenerative condition occurring within the vascular tree and resulting in occlusion and/or loss of elasticity of the vessel.

ATP, ADP, AMP   High-energy compounds important in energy metabolism.

Autoimmunity   Immunity developed to self-antigens.

B-cells   Lymphocytes produced by the bone marrow that produce antibodies. B-cells kill foreign cells "at a distance," while T-cells must be in contact with the foreigner to kill it.

β cells   Insulin-producing cells in the pancreas.

Bacteriophage   Bacteria eating.

Bariatric surgeon   A physician who specializes in the surgical treatment of obesity.

Basal metabolism   The minimum amount of energy needed by the body at rest and in the fasting (not starving) state.

BMI   Body mass index; used as an indicator of body fatness. Not applicable to people with large muscle mass such as competitive athletes.

Bradycardia	Slow heartbeat.
Buffer	A compound that resists changes in pH.
Bulimia	Self-induced vomiting.
Cachexia	Tissue wasting.
Cancer	A group of diseases characterized by an uncontrolled growth of a certain cell type.
Carcinogenesis	The process of developing cancer.
Cariogenesis	The process of tooth decay.
Catabolic reactions	Reactions that result in the breakdown of large molecules to small ones.
Catecholamines	Neurotransmitters (epinephrine, norepinephrine, and dopamine) that orchestrate the fight-or-flight response to danger.
Cations	Molecules having a positive charge.
Cecum	A blind appendage of the intestinal tract located at the juncture of the small and large intestine. Also called the *appendix*.
Cell-mediated immunity	Immunity resulting from direct interaction with antigen-specific T-cells.
Chloride shift	Part of the system that maintains the blood acid–base balance. Chloride and bicarbonate ions exchange across the red cell membrane.
Cholecystitis	Inflammation of the gall bladder.
Cholesterol	A steroid synthesized by the body that serves as the beginning substance for the synthesis of a variety of other essential constituents.
Chyle	A turbid white or yellow fluid taken up by the lacteals as part of the process of lipid absorption.
Chyme	The semi-fluid mass of partially digested food extruded from the stomach into the small intestine.
Colon	Large intestine.
Cortex	In a two-part organ such as the adrenal gland, the cortex is in the middle while the medulla is on the outside.
Creatine phosphate	A high-energy compound found in muscle.
Cytokines	A family of small peptide hormones produced and released by macrophages, adipose tissue, brain, and so forth. Leptin is a cytokine.

Cytosol   Cell sap; what is left in the cell after the formed organelles (nucleus, mitochondria, endoplasmic reticulum, peroxisomes, microsomes, etc.) are removed.

Cytotoxic agents   Materials that destroy cells.

Degrade   To reduce large molecules to smaller ones.

Dermatitis   Inflammation of the skin.

DEXA   Dual energy x-ray densitometry; a method used to determine bone density and also body fatness.

Diabetes mellitus   A large group of genetic diseases characterized by the body's inability to use glucose appropriately.

Diffusion   A uniform distribution of solutes on both sides of a membrane.

Distal   Away from the center of the body.

Distention   Expansion above normal.

Diuresis   Urine excretion in excess of normal.

Diuretics   Drugs that promote the excretion of water in the urine.

Duodenum   The first one-third of the small intestine.

Edema   Excess water accumulation in the body particularly in the hands and feet.

Electrolytes   Molecules that have either a positive or negative charge.

Embryo   The initial stage of development of a fertilized egg.

Emulsion   A mixture of fat and water held together by a substance that has both hydrophilic and lipophilic properties.

Endocytosis   The process of forming a vesicle within the secreting cell.

Enterocytes   The absorptive cells lining the intestinal tract.

Etiology   The study of the cause of disease.

Eukaryote   Complex, multicellular organism.

Eupnea   Normal breathing.

Extracellular   Outside the cell.

Feces   Material excreted from the anus; undigested food and unused digestive material.

Fetus   An unborn child.

Fibroblasts   Progenitor cells that can differentiate into more specific cell types.

Flatulence   Release of gases from the anus.

GABA   Gamma amino butyric acid, a neurotransmitter that quiets excited neurons.

Gastrin	A small peptide that stimulates the release of hydrochloric acid by the parietal cells of the stomach.
Gene	A fragment of the DNA that carries information about a specific protein the cell can make.
Genotype	The inherited characteristics of an animal or cell.
Geophagia	Dirt eating.
Glomerulus	The filtration unit of the kidney.
Glucagon	Hormone released by the pancreatic islet cells that counteracts the action of insulin.
Gluconeogenesis	Synthesis of glucose from noncarbohydrate precursors.
Glycogenesis	Synthesis of glycogen.
Glycogenolysis	Breakdown of glycogen.
Glycolysis	Catabolism of glucose.
HANES (NHANES)	Health and Nutrition Examination Survey sponsored by the U.S. Centers for Disease Control, a unit of the U.S. Public Health Service.
Hematocrit	The volume of erythrocytes packed by centrifugation in a given volume of blood.
Hematopoiesis	The synthesis of red blood cells.
Heme	The protein portion of hemoglobin that holds iron.
Hemoglobin	The iron-containing protein in red blood cells.
Hypercorticolism	Excess levels of cortisol in the blood; characteristic of Cushing's syndrome.
Hyperinsulinemia	Excess levels of insulin in the blood; a characteristic of insulin resistance by the insulin target tissues.
Hyperkalemia	Excess levels of potassium in the blood.
Hyperlipidemia	Excess levels of lipids in the blood.
Hypernatremia	Excess levels of sodium in the blood.
Hyperphagia	Overeating; eating far more food than the body requires to sustain good health and a normal body weight.
Hypertension	Higher than normal blood pressure.
Hyperthermia	Higher than normal body temperature.
Hypertrophy	Increased cell size or organ size.
Hypocalcemia	Below normal levels of calcium in the blood.
Hypoglycemia	Below normal levels of glucose in the blood (lower than 80 mg/dL).
Hypokalemia	Below normal levels of potassium in the blood.

Hyponatremia	Below normal levels of sodium in the blood.
Hypoproteinemia	Below normal levels of protein in the blood.
Hypotension	Below normal blood pressure.
Hypothermia	Below normal body temperature.
Hypothyroidism	Below normal levels of thyroid hormone levels in the blood.
Hypovolemia	Below normal blood volume.
Ileum	The last one-third of the small intestine.
Insulin	Hormone released by the pancreatic islet cells; promotes glucose use.
Intercellular	Between cells.
Interstitial fluid	Fluids between cells.
Intracellular	Within the cell.
Intravascular	Within the vascular system.
Ion	An element with either a positive or negative charge.
Ischemia	Impaired blood flow causing oxygen and nutrient deprivation.
Jejunum	The middle one-third of the small intestine.
Labile	Easily degraded; unstable.
Leptin	A cytokine released by the adipose tissue that signals satiety to the brain.
Lipogenesis	Synthesis of fatty acids and fat.
Lipolysis	Breakdown (catabolism) of lipids.
Lumen	Interior aspect of a vessel.
Lymphokines (Interleukins 1–12)	Cytokines produced by the lymphocytes.
Macronutrient	Large molecules of nutritional value. These are the carbohydrates, fats, and proteins.
Macrophages	Large mononuclear cells that phagositize foreign compounds and neutralize them.
MCV	Mean corpuscular volume.
MHC	Major histocompatibility complex, molecules that help the lymphocytes identify foreign materials as antigens.
Class I MHC proteins	Antigen-presenting molecules found on all nucleated cells.
Class II MHC proteins	Antigen-presenting molecules found on macrophages and B-cells.

Micelles	Small particles of lipid and bile salts where the water-soluble portion is on the outside and the lipid-soluble portion is on the inside.
Micronutrients	Small molecules of nutritional importance. These include the essential minerals and vitamins.
Milliequivalent (mEq)	A measurement of the concentration of electrolytes in solution. It is determined by multiplying the milligrams of solute per liter by the valence of the solute divided by the molecular weight of the solute.
Morbidity	Illness leading to death.
Mortality	Cause of death.
Myocyte	Muscle cell.
Obesity	Excess fat stores.
Olfaction	Sense of smell.
Oliguria	Decreased urine production.
Oocyte	Egg produced by the ovary.
Orthostatic hypotension	Hypotension that results from standing for too long in a tense position.
Osmosis	The passage of solvents across a membrane so that the number of solute molecules is equal on each side.
Osteoblasts	Bone-forming cells.
Osteoclasts	Cells responsible for bone remodeling.
Osteomalacia	Softening of the bone through loss of bone mineral.
Osteopenia	Decreased bone mass.
Osteoporosis	Demineralization of the bone resulting in a fragile porous bone.
Oxidation	Removal of electrons using oxygen as the electron acceptor.
Passive diffusion	A process for the movement of solutes across a membrane without the use of either a carrier or energy.
Passive immunity	Acquisition of immunity through the transfer of antibodies into the body.
Peritonitis	Inflammation of the peritoneal (abdominal) cavity.
Perturbation	A disturbance from normal.
pH	The numerical representation of the hydrogen ion concentration in a solution. The range is from 1 to 14. A pH of 1 is very acidic; a pH of 14 is very alkaline.

Phenotype	The physical characteristics of an individual as determined by the individual's genotype.
Plasma	The fluid left from blood after the formed elements have been removed.
Polydipsea	Greater than normal thirst and water consumption.
Polyuria	Greater than normal urine production and release.
Postprandial	After a meal.
Prokaryote	Single-cell organism.
Proton	A particle in the nucleus of an atom with a positive charge.
Proximal	Toward the center of the body.
RBC	Red blood cell.
Receptor	A general term applied to any protein in any part of the body that binds to a specific compound and allows it to do its job.
RER	Rough endoplasmic reticulum, an organelle in the cell used for the storage/release of regulatory components.
Ribosome	An organelle in the cell where protein synthesis takes place.
Sarcolemma	Membrane surrounding the muscle unit.
Sarcomere	Muscle unit.
Sarcoplasm	Fluid within the muscle unit.
Sarcoplasmic reticulum	An organelle in the cell; it is a fine network of membranous sacs within the muscle unit. Calcium and other important regulatory molecules are stored here only to be released when the muscle is signaled to contract.
Satiety	A sense of being satisfied that enough food has been consumed.
Serum	The blood fluid after the clotting factors and red cells have been removed.
Sex-linked traits	Traits carried on either the X or Y chromosome.
Stable isotope	A nonradioactive isotope.
Stool	Feces.
Supine	Lying on one's back.
Symptoms	Indications of disease.
Syncytial, syncytium	A multinucleated mass formed by the secondary union of originally separate cells.

T-cells	Lymphocytes produced by the thymus gland.
Killer T-cells	Lymphocytes that in contact with an infected cell kill the cell.
Helper T-cells	Lymphocytes that regulate the activity of B-cells.
Suppressor T-cells	Lymphocytes that suppress the activity of B-cells.
Tachycardia	Rapid heartbeat.
Thermogenesis	The production and release of heat.

Index

A

Acquired immune deficiency syndrome (AIDS), 50, 93
Active transport, 67, 71
Adaptation, 13
Age and nutrition, 121–126
  age effects on metabolic pathways, 123
  age-related changes in metabolism, 123–124
  age-related impaired mental functions, 121
  aging process, 121–123
  case study
    elderly tiredness, 125
    palpitations, 126
  hormone changes with age, 124
  insulin, peripheral cell responsivity to, 124
  lipids, age-related changes, 124
  senescence, 121
AIDS, *see* Acquired immune deficiency syndrome
Allergic reactions, 95
Allergies, 96
Amino acid absorption, 69
Aminopeptidase, 68
Anabolism, 139
Anasakis, 106
Anemia, 43–48
  aspirin and, 122
  causes of, 43–46
  iron deficiency without, 46
  non-nutritional anemia, 48
  normal blood values for measurements made to assess presence of, 47
  other nutrients and anemia, 47
  pharmacological treatment of iron deficiency, 46
  toxicology of iron overload, 46–47
Anorexia, 23
Antibodies
  IgE, 95
  IgG, 16
  IgM, 16
  structure, 95
Antigens, 93, 95
Appendix, 141
Arteriosclerosis, 12

Aspirin
  anemia and, 122
  platelet activity and, 50
Atherosclerosis, 12
Atrial-ventricle (A-V) node, 128
Autoimmune diseases, 12, 96
A-V node, *see* Atrial-ventricle node

B

Bacteria, 103–105
Bariatric surgery, 32
Basal energy need, learning activity, 131
Basal metabolic rate (BMR), 30
B-cells, 94, 95
Bile acids, primary, 73
Bile salts, 72
Biochemical individuality, 81
Blood, 43–56
  aspirin, platelet activity and, 50
  baseline measurements, 14
  blood clotting, 49–50
  blood components, 44
  blood groups, 48
  blood pressure, 51–52
  blood pressure under hormonal control, 51
  case study
    automobile accident, 54
    pioneer women (late 1800s), 55
    vegetarianism, 56
  causes of nutritional anemia, 43–48
    non-nutritional anemia, 48
    other nutrients and anemia, 47
    pharmacological treatment of iron deficiency, 46
    toxicology of iron overload, 46–47
  clot formation, 49
  cobalt, 47
  constituents, 6
  copper, 47
  diuretics, 52
  erythropoiesis, 43
  hematopoiesis, 43
  high blood pressure, 51

hypertension, 51
iron deficiency without anemia, 46
iron uptake and loss, 45
lead poisoning, 48
learning activity, nutritional status, 53
menstruation, iron loss with, 45, 46
normal values for, 6
nutrients needed for red cell production, 44
replacement cells, 43
Rh factor, 48
values, assessment of presence of anemia, 47
vascular system, 43
vitamins, 47
white cells, 50
BMR, *see* Basal metabolic rate
Body weight regulation, 30–33
    bariatric surgery, 32–33
    diet products, 31–32
    drugs in treatment of obesity, 31
    treatment of obesity, 30–31
Bones, stones and, 111–119
    bladder stones, 116
    bone mineralization, 111
    calciomimetic agents, 114
    calcium
        -binding protein, 112
        GI absorption of, 111
    case study
        becoming shorter, 117
        hip fracture, 119
        pain, 118
    cystine, 116
    gouty nephropathy, 116
    hormones affecting bone formation and
        remodeling, 112
    hydroxyapatite, 111
    hyperparathyroidism, 114
    metabolic bone diseases, 111, 112
    nutrients important to bone health, 113
    osteomalacia, 111, 114
    osteopenia, 114
    osteoporosis, 111, 113
    other bone diseases, 114–115
    oxaluria, 115
    Paget's disease, 114
    remodeling, 111
    renal osteodystrophy, 114
    renal stone disease, 115
    skeletal problems associated with renal disease, 114
    skeleton composition, 113
    types of stones, 115–116
    weak estrogens, 113
Brucella, 105
Bulimia, 23

C

Calciomimetic agents, 114
Calcium, 27–28
    absorption, vitamin D and, 111–112
    -binding protein, 112
    GI absorption of, 111
    inadequate intake, 27
    muscle and, 128
    muscle contraction and, 25
    in skeleton, 111
Camplobacterium contamination, 105
Carbohydrate
    absorption, active transport, 71
    digestion, 69–70
Case study
    Africa, 89
    alcoholic, 65
    analysis, 3
    answers to problems, 3
    Army, 138
    automobile accident, 54
    baby, 40–41, 77
    becoming shorter, 117
    cat, 101
    concentration camp, 42
    cyclist, 135
    definition of, 1–2
    dog, 100
    elderly tiredness, 125
    epidemiological, 16–19
        background, 17–19
        conclusion, 19
        story, 16–17
    food supplements, 78
    gaining weight, 35–36
    gastric analysis, 75
    gastric bypass, 38–39
    gastrointestinal problems, 102
    goldfish, 37
    heart attack, 137
    heart trouble, 79–80
    hip fracture, 119
    intestinal virus, 110
    key words and meanings, 3
    light intensity, 64
    milk
    organic farming, 109
    organization of information, 4
    pain, 76, 118
    palpitations, 126
    parakeet, 99
    pioneer women (late 1800s), 55
    professional football, 136
    relevant literature, 3–4
    scurvy, 66
    summary preparation, 4
    traveler's illness, 107–108
    type 2 diabetes, 91–92
    vegetarianism, 56
CBC, *see* Complete blood count
CDC, *see* Centers for Disease Control
Cell apoptosis, 129

Centers for Disease Control (CDC), 15, 103
Central nervous system (CNS), 24
Chloride, 26–27
Cholecystectomy, 73
Cholecystokinin, 68, 72
Cholesterol levels, elevated, 11
Chromosomes, 81
Chronic disease, 11
Chyme, 68
Clinical assessments, normal laboratory values for, 7
Clinical terms, meanings, 4
Clostridium botulinum, 105
CNS, *see* Central nervous system
Cobalt, 47
Colipase, 72
Colon, intussusception of, 110
Complete blood count (CBC), 62
Congenital diseases, 13
Copper, 47
Coronary vessel disease, 11
Coumarin, 49
Cytokines, 94

D

Degenerative diseases, 11, 13
DEXA, *see* Dual energy x-ray absorptiometry
Diabesity, 85
Diabetes, 85, 91
Diacylglycerol, 72
Diet histories, 59
Dipeptidase, 68
Diphyllobothrium, 106
Disease(s), 11–19
    arteriosclerosis, 12
    atherosclerosis, 12
    autoimmune diseases, 12, 96
    bone, 111, 112
    causes of disease, 12–13
    chronic disease, 11
    congenital diseases, 13
    definition of disease, 11–12
    degenerative diseases, 11, 13
    duration of disease, 14–15
    epidemic, 12
    epidemiological approach to disease
        management, 15
    etiology, 11, 12–13
    genetic, 83
    genetic factors, 11
    histopathology, 12
    homeostasis, 11
    idiopathic diseases, 12
    IgG antibodies, 16
    IgM antibodies, 16
    incidence rate, 12
    infectious disease, 12–13
    joints and connective tissue, 122
    keeping track of disease, 12

    laboratory work, 13–14
    metabolic bone disease, 111
    mortality, 12
    pathophysiology, 11, 12
    plaque, 11
    prevalence, 12
    risk factors, 13
    sex-linked genetic disease, 84
    signs and symptoms, 13
    study of disease, 12
    tissues used for laboratory assessment, 14
    zoonotic diseases, 93
Diuretics, 52
DNA
    description of, 81
    function of, 82
    muscle disorders, 130
Dual energy x-ray absorptiometry (DEXA), 14, 102, 117
Duchenne muscular dystrophy, 130

E

Effectors, 22
Eicosanoids, 43
Elastase, 68
Electrolyte(s), 44
    balance, hormones and, 51
    imbalance, 23, 25, 122
    loss, 25
    major extracellular, 25
    major intracellular, 26
    muscle contraction and, 28
    passive diffusion, 67
Endopeptidases, 68
Epidemiological case study, 16–19
    background, 17–19
    conclusion, 19
    story, 16–17
Epidemiologists, 12
Erythropoiesis, 43
Escherichia coli, 103
Etiology of disease, 11
Eukaryotic contaminants (molds and parasites), 106
Exopeptidases, 68

F

Fat absorption, bile acids and, 73
Ferritin, 43, 45, 85
FFQ, *see* Food frequency questionnaire
Fight-or-ight response, 22
Food-borne illness, prevention of, 106, *see also*
        Health, food and
Food choices, 57–66
    albumin levels, 62
    case study
        alcoholic, 65
        light intensity, 64
        scurvy, 66

detoxification reactions, 63
dietary guidelines, 57
diet assessment, 57–61
diet histories, 59
food record method, 58
gender differences, 62
hemoglobin levels, 62
laboratory tests, 62–63
malnutrition, physical signs of, 60
MyPyramid, 57
nutrient intake, estimation of, 58
nutritional assessment, 61–62
observation method, 59
product labels, 58
24-hour recall, 57–58
vitamin/mineral supplements, 61
Web sites for food intake information, 58
Food diary, 34
Food frequency questionnaire (FFQ), 58, 59
Food production, cleanliness in, 106
Food safety, *see* Health, food and
Food utilization, 67–80
absorption, 67
active transport, 67, 71
amino acid absorption, 69
aminopeptidase, 68
bile acids, primary, 73
bile salts, 72
carbohydrate absorption, 71
carbohydrate digestion, 69–70
case study
baby, 77
food supplements, 78
gastric analysis, 75
heart trouble, 79–80
pain, 76
cholecystectomy, 73
cholecystokinin, 68, 72
chyme, 68
colipase, 72
diacylglycerol, 72
dipeptidase, 68
elastase, 68
endopeptidases, 68
exopeptidases, 68
facilitated diffusion, 67
fat absorption, bile acids and, 73
fatty acids, 73
fructose, 71
gallstones, 73
Golgi complex, 74
lactose intolerance, 70
leucocytosis, 76
lipid digestion and absorption, 71–74
lipid esterase, 72
micelles, 72, 73
milk fat, 72
mobile glucose transporters, 71
monosaccharides, 71

passive diffusion, 67
pepsin, 68
peptidases, categories, 68
protein digestion, 68–69
protein digestive enzymes, 68
retrieval of nutrients from food, 67
sodium-dependent transporter, 71
trypsin, 68
Fructose, 71

G

Gallstones, 73
Gastric bypass, 32, 38–39
Gastrointestinal (GI) absorption, 111
Genetics, 81–92
age-related changes in serum lipids, 124
amino acids, 82
appetite-suppressing signal, 85
biochemical individuality, 81
case study
Africa, 89
milk
type 2 diabetes, 91–02
cell division, 83
chromosomes, 81
diabesity, 85
diabetes, 85
disease and, 11
diseases of autosomal recessive type, 83
DNA
description of, 81
function of, 82
ferritin synthesis, 85
gene–nutrient interactions, 84
genes, genotype, and phenotype, 81–83
genome, 81
genotype, 82
heterozygote, 83
homozygote, 83
how environment shapes phenotypic expression
of genotype, 84–87
how we inherit genotype and phenotype, 83–84
insulin resistance, 85
learning activity, family tree, 88
mutation, 82, 83
NADP-linked xylitol dehydrogenase, 82
nutrients affecting translation, 86
obesity, risk factors with, 86
OXPHOS system characteristics, 84
phenotype, 82
polymorphism, 82
protein synthesis, 83
sex-linked genetic disease, 84
sex-linked mutation, 84
uncoupling proteins, 85
vitamin K deficiency, 86
World War II food rationing, 85
Yemenite Jews, 84

Genome, 81
GI absorption, *see* Gastrointestinal absorption
Glossary, 139–147
Glucose, 69
Gouty nephropathy, 116

H

Health, food and, 103–110
    case study
        intestinal virus, 110
        organic farming, 109
        traveler's illness, 107–108
    Escherichia coli, 103
    food-borne pathogens, 103–106
        bacteria, 103–105
        eukaryotic contaminants, 104, 106
        molds, 104, 106
        parasites, 104, 106
        viruses, 105, 110
    food safety, 103
    intussusception of colon, 110
    pathogens causing food-borne illness, 104
    prevention, 106
    recognition, 106
Health organizations, Web sites, 2
Heart disease, death from, 130
Helicobacter pylori, 105
Hematopoiesis, 43
High blood pressure, 51
Histopathology, 12
Homeostasis, 11, 21–42
    adaptation, 13
    anorexia, 23
    basal energy expenditure, 30
    body weight regulation, 30–33
        bariatric surgery, 32–33
        diet products, 31–32
        drugs in treatment of obesity, 31
        treatment of obesity, 30–31
    bulimia, 23
    case study
        baby, 40–41
        concentration camp, 42
        gaining weight, 35–36
        gastric bypass, 38–39
        goldfish, 37
    chloride shift, 26
    definition of, 21
    effectors, 22
    fatness, 29
    fight-or--ight response, 22
    gastric bypass, 32, 38–39
    hyperphagia, 28
    hypocalcemia, 28
    lactose-free diet, 24
    laxatives, chronic use of, 28
    lazy fish, 23
    lean body mass, maintenance of, 30

learning activity, food diary, 34
leptin, 29
lipase inhibitors, 31
liposuction, 32
low-fat diet, 24
magnesium deficiency, 28
malnourishment, 23
malnutrition, 24–28
    calcium, 27–28
    chloride, 26–27
    magnesium, 28
    potassium, 26
    sodium, 25
neurotransmitters, 22
other instances of homeostatic regulation, 28–30
    growth and development, 28
    obesity, 28–30
oxygen consumption and carbon dioxide
        release, 23
physiology of nutrition and, 23–24
protein-calorie malnutrition, 25
protein-energy malnutrition, 25
receptors, 22
regulation of, 21–23
set-point theory, 30
sodium-calcium antiport system, 25
sodium-potassium ATPase, 25
Hormone(s), 43
    age-related changes, 124
    bone formation, 112
    electrolyte balance and, 51
Hydroxyapatite, 111
Hyperparathyroidism, 114
Hyperphagia, 28
Hypertension, 51

I

Idiopathic diseases, 12
IFN, *see* Interferon
IgE antibodies, 95
IgG antibodies, 16
IgM antibodies, 16
IL, *see* Interleukins
Immune system
    diseases, 96–97
    functioning of, 93–95
Immunization procedures, 95
Infectious disease, 12–13
Information, organization of (case study), 4
Insulin
    –glucose relationship, aging and, 123
    peripheral cell responsivity to, 124
    resistance, 85
Interferon (IFN), 94
Interleukins (IL), 94
Intussusception of colon, 110
Iron deficiency, 46

L

Lactase, 69, 70
Lactose
    -free diet, 24
    intolerance, 70
Laxatives, chronic use of, 28
Lazy fish, 23
Lead poisoning, 48
Lean body mass, maintenance of, 30
Learning activity
    activity cost, 132–133
    basal energy need, 131
    epidemiological case study, 16–19
    family tree, 88
    food diary, 34
    medical terms
        meanings, 9
        prefixes, 8
    nutritional status, 53
    performance-enhancing products, 134
Legionella pneumophila, 16
Leptin, 29
Leucocytosis, 76
Lipase inhibitors, 31
Lipid(s)
    age-related changes, 124
    digestion and absorption, 71–74
    esterase, 72
Liposuction, 32
Low-fat diet, 24

M

Mad cow disease, 93
Magnesium, 28
Major histocompatibility proteins, 94
Malignant hyperthermia, 130
Malnourishment, 23
Malnutrition, 24–28
    calcium, 27–28
    chloride, 26–27
    chronic, 25
    geriatric, 121
    magnesium, 28
    menstruation and, 61
    muscle and, 129
    physical signs of, 60
    potassium, 26
    predisposing conditions, 61
    sodium, 25
Maltase, 70
Maltose, 69
Medical terms, prefixes used in, 5
Memory cells, 95
Menstruation
    iron loss with, 45, 46
    malnutrition and, 61
Metabolic bone disease, 111, 112

Metabolic –ux, 43
Micelles, 72, 73
Milk
    fat, 72
    fatty acids, 73
    raw, contaminant of, 105
Mineral absorption, 74
Mobile glucose transporters, 71
Molds, 104, 106
Monosaccharides, 71
Muscle, 127–138
    calcium, 128
    cell apoptosis, 129
    contraction, sodium and, 25
    depolarizationflrepolarization, 27
    Duchenne muscular dystrophy, 130
    heart disease, death from, 130
    malignant hyperthermia, 130
    muscular dystrophy, 130
    myocytes, 127
    sarcomere, 127
    sarcoplasm, 127
    soft pork, 130
    striated muscle, 127
Muscular dystrophy, 130
Myocytes, 127
MyPyramid, 57

N

NADP-linked xylitol dehydrogenase, 82
National Health and Nutrition Examination Survey
        (NHANES), 61
Neurotransmitters, 22
NHANES, *see* National Health and Nutrition
        Examination Survey

O

Obesity
    cultural in–uences, 29
    genetic susceptibility to, 11
    hyperphagia, 28
    morbid, 39
    phenotypes, 85
    risk factors with, 86
    treatment of, 30
Orlistat, 31
Osteomalacia, 111
Osteopenia, 114
Osteoporosis, 111
Oxaluria, 115
OXPHOS system characteristics, 84

P

Paget's disease, 114
Parasites, 104, 106
Parathyroid hormone (PTH), 112

Passive diffusion, 67
Pathophysiology, 12
PCM, *see* Protein-calorie malnutrition
Pepsin, 68
Peptidases, categories, 68
Performance-enhancing products, 134
Pets and people, 93–102
    allergic reactions, 95, 96
    amino acid sequences, antigens and, 95
    antibodies, 95
    antigens, 93, 94, 95
    autoimmune disease, 96
    B-cells, 94, 95
    case study
        cat, 101
        dog, 100
        gastrointestinal problems, 102
        horse, 98
        parakeet, 99
    colony stimulation factors, 94
    cytokines, 94
    how immune system works, 93–95
    immune system diseases, 96–97
    immunization procedures, 95
    interferons, 94
    interleukins, 94
    major histocompatibility proteins, 94
    memory cells, 95
    self-proteins, 96
    suppressor T-cell, 95
    systemic lupus erythematosus, 97
    T-helper cells, 94
    tumor necrosis factor, 94
    zoonotic diseases, 93
Plaque, 11
Pneumonia, 18
Potassium, 26, 52
Protein(s)
    autoimmune disease, 97
    calcium-binding protein, 112
    -calorie malnutrition (PCM), 25
    digestion, 68–69
    digestive enzymes, 68
    -energy malnutrition, 25
    major histocompatibility proteins, 94
    self-proteins, 96
    synthesis
        age-related decline in, 124
        genetics and, 83
    uncoupling, 85
PTH, *see* Parathyroid hormone
Pyridoxine deficiency, reversal of, 14

R

Receptors, 22
Renal disease, skeletal problems associated
        with, 114
Renal osteodystrophy, 114

Renal stone disease, 115
Rh factor, 48
Risk factors (disease), 13

S

Salmonella contamination, 105
Sarcomere, 127
Scurvy, 66, 113
Self-proteins, 96
Senescence, 121
Set-point theory, 30
Sex-linked genetic disease, 84
Sex-linked mutation, 84
Shellfish, raw, 105
Shigella contamination, 105
Skeletal muscle, 127
Sodium, 25
    blood pressure and, 52
    -calcium antiport system, 25
    -dependent transporter, 71
    -potassium ATPase, 25
Soft pork, 130
Staphylococcus aureus, 105
Stones, *see* Bones, stones and
Sucrase, 70
Suppressor T-cell, 95
Systemic lupus erythematosus, 97

T

Taenia, 106
T-helper cells, 94
Thyroid hormone production, age-related declines
        in, 124
TNF, *see* Tumor necrosis factor
Transferrin, 43
Trichinella, 106
Trypsin, 68
Tumor necrosis factor (TNF), 94

U

UCPs, *see* Uncoupling proteins
Uncoupling proteins (UCPs), 85

V

Vascular system, 43, *see also* Blood
Vegetarianism, 56
Vibrio-related illness, 105
Viruses, 105, 110
Vitamin(s)
    absorption, 74
    bone and, 113
    supplements, 61

vitamin D, calcium absorption and, 111–112
vitamin deficiency, anemia and, 47
vitamin K
  blood clotting and, 49
  deficiency, 86
Vomiting, self-induced, 35

W

Weak estrogens, 113
Web sites
  food intake information, 58
  Health organizations, 2
WIC, *see* Women, Infants, and Children program

Women, Infants, and Children program (WIC), 57
World War II food rationing, 85

X

Xenecal, 31

Y

Yersinia contamination, 105

Z

Zoonotic diseases, 93